POULTRY HOMEOPATHY

"Advancing Homeopathic Research in Poultry Healthcare"

2nd Edition

DR MUHAMMED KS

BlueRose ONE
Stories Matter
NewDelhi • London

BLUEROSE PUBLISHERS
India | U.K.

BlueRose ONE
Stories Matter
NewDelhi • London

For permissions requests or inquiries regarding this publication, please contact:

BLUEROSE PUBLISHERS
www.BlueRoseONE.com
info@bluerosepublishers.com
+91 8882 898 898
+4407342408967

ISBN: 978-93-6261-642-5

Cover design: Tahira
Typesetting: Tanya Raj Upadhyay

First Edition: July 2024

PREFACE

Homeopathy medicines in poultry are getting popularized because of its quick and prompt action. Poultry farming in India has registered phenomenal growth during last two and half decades and India ranks second in Egg Production and fifth in meat production in the world. Homeopathy medicines works quite efficiently in the treatment of the poultry diseases over and above they are economical, easy to administer, safe and have quick action. Intensive raising of poultry in commercial poultry farming, inevitably exposes the flock to various diseases causing mortality and loss of production. Homeopathy remedies can cover wide range for infectious, non-infectious diseases, metabolic and nutritional disorders as well as behavioral and environmental disorders in poultry.

With increasing antibiotics uses which poses antimicrobial resistance to it and hence world facing challenges as antibiotics either banned or used with strict regulations. Homeopathy provides a viable alternative therapy for disease management in poultry as it's an economical and safer to use. It has demonstrated its pivotal role in anti-viral management and increasing awareness for the use of homeopathy in poultry paves the way for One Health Approach working with the goal of achieving optimal health outcomes, recognizing the interconnection between people, animals, plants, and their shared environment.

This book will provide insight for the use of such remedies as an easily understandable ways and means for the poultry industry. The author has intended to make use of such alternative therapy with inclusion of the merits of the homeopathy medicines after studied with the scientific background and it will serve as reference book for poultry keepers and industry as a whole.

Dr. R. S. Joshi
Professor and Head
Livestock Farm Complex
Veterinary College
Kamdhenu University Anand, Gujarat

FOREWORD

Poultry farming is a major industry across the globe that provides an important source of nutrition and livelihood for millions. However, poultry health issues like infectious diseases can devastate flocks and cause major economic losses. This highlights the need for effective, safe and sustainable approaches to poultry healthcare.

As the world continues to evolve and innovate, so does our understanding of healthcare. This evolution extends to every corner of medicine, including veterinary care. The second edition of "Poultry Homoeopathy - Advancing Homoeopathic Research in Poultry Health care" by Dr. Muhammed KS is a testament to this evolution.

Dr. Muhammed KS, a distinguished expert in the field, brings a wealth of knowledge and experience to this book. The primary focus is on the homoeopathic approach to poultry diseases, with the aim of enhancing poultry health and research through the homoeopathic perspective.

In this edition, Dr. Muhammed KS delves into the source and evolution of veterinary homoeopathy, highlighting its scope and potential in poultry research. The book also covers essential topics like routes of drug administration, drug dosage forms, and the role of homoeopathy in poultry farming.

In this extensively revised Second Edition of "Poultry Homoeopathy", Dr. Muhammed K.S. draws from his extensive clinical expertise to illustrate the principles and practice of using homoeopathy to prevent and manage key poultry diseases. The book explains homoeopathic philosophy and concepts, drug administration methods, research parameters along with classification and homoeopathic management of major poultry diseases. Enriched with clinical experiences and new topics, it aims to advance homoeopathic research and application in the poultry industry.

I am confident that second revised edition of this book will be a valuable addition to the library of any poultry farmer, veterinarian, or homoeopathy enthusiast. It not only provides a comprehensive overview of homoeopathy's role in poultry health but also offers practical advice and quick remedies for common issues.

I congratulate Dr. Muhammed KS on this outstanding work and wish him continued success in advancing homoeopathic research in poultry health care. Integrating mainstream poultry healthcare with such complementary approaches can pave the way for better poultry health, reduced antibiotic usage and a more sustainable industry.

Dr. Mansoor Ali KR
Professor & HOD
Govt Homoeopathic Medical College Calicut
Chief Advisor: Homeobook.com

FOREWORD

As the State President of the Indian Homeopathic Medical Association (IHMA) Kerala, it is with great enthusiasm that I introduce this seminal research book exploring the scope of homeopathy in poultry healthcare.

In recent years, the poultry industry has undergone rapid expansion to meet the growing demand for poultry products. However, this expansion has brought with it numerous challenges, including disease outbreaks, antibiotic resistance, and concerns about animal welfare. In this context, homeopathy emerges as a promising alternative approach to promote the health and well-being of poultry.

Homeopathy, with its emphasis on individualized treatment and gentle yet effective remedies, holds tremendous potential in addressing the unique healthcare needs of poultry. By harnessing the principles of similia similibus curentur (like cures like) and potentization, homeopathic veterinarians can provide holistic solutions that not only alleviate symptoms but also enhance the overall vitality and resilience of poultry flocks.

This book showcases the latest research and practical applications of homeopathy in poultry healthcare. From managing common ailments like respiratory infections and gastrointestinal disorders to improving growth rates and egg production, the contributions of our esteemed researchers shed light on the diverse ways in which homeopathy can benefit the poultry industry.

As we strive towards sustainable and ethical practices in animal husbandry, homeopathy offers a compelling avenue for promoting health and productivity in poultry without resorting to excessive antibiotic use or other harmful interventions. By embracing this integrative approach, we can create healthier environments for both animals and humans alike.

I extend my sincere appreciation to the authors, researchers, and practitioners who have contributed to this book. May their insights inspire further exploration and innovation in the field of homeopathic poultry healthcare, ultimately leading to healthier and more resilient poultry populations.

Warm regards,

Dr. Mohammed Shameem
State President
Indian Homeopathic Medical Association (IHMA)

FOREWORD

Veterinary Homoeopathy, though an up and coming Science, will hold an important place in Veterinary Science in the near future. While preliminary research has proven efficiency and scope of this new branch, a lot of work is still required, to mainstream the integration of Homoeopathy into animal husbandry and Veterinary Science, in general.

This is where Dr. Muhammed K. S' latest work, 'Poultry Homoeopathy,' will be deemed beneficial to both Homoeopaths and Veterinarians alike. Having personally seen him strive hard for the past few years to perfect his findings and research on this novel topic, I am extremely glad to see him finally launch this work to the public.

Unlike Homoeopathy for human beings, Poultry Homoeopathy does come with its fair share of challenges, the most important being the difficulty to collect symptoms. Unlike communicating humans, animals aren't able to express their symptoms very efficiently. Thus, it goes without saying that, it not only takes an in-depth knowledge of Homoeopathy, but, also a deep understanding of the animal Anatomy, Physiology and other allied subjects, to embark on a journey to master Poultry Homoeopathy. This could very well be one reason why many physicians have shied away from this topic.

A Homoeopath, by degree, Dr. Mohammed K. S, embarked on this journey a few years ago, and through painstaking research, both literature and lab-based, he is out with his surprising findings. His findings have very wonderfully been presented in this work.

I hope and pray that, this work by Dr. Mohammed K. S becomes a precursor to further advanced findings, that subsequently make Homoeopathy the preferred mode of treatment in Veterinary clinics and hospitals world over. We humans have enjoyed the "rapid, gentle and permanent" cure that Homoeopathy provides, for close to two centuries now. Being the caretakers of this world, let us now pass on these benefits to our companions, the animals!

Dr. Sudhi.TK, BSc (Zoology), BHMS
Chief Physician – KHCH

FOREWORD

The process of writing is replete with complexities. Ensuring that the content is expressed with finesse of language is not easy. Maintaining the structure and the lucidity of thought is a huge challenge.

A book on Homoeopathy and that too a book on Homoeopathic approach to poultry diseases as well as scope and advantages of homoeopathy in the field of poultry research and treatment can be wrought with many more challenges. Although it's an age-old tested field of Science, the availability of research material is always a question mark.

That's why when an attempt is made to delve deep into understanding, interpreting, explaining & prescribing this ancient filed of knowledge, it’s an admirable act.

In this book the effort to cover the Infectious and parasitic diseases attacking Poultry, Metabolic and nutritional disorders connected with poultry, its management and prevention with Homoeopathic system is highly commendable. This will be an asset to Humanity.

I congratulate Dr Mohammad K S on the painstaking compilation of facts, figures and anecdotes. The book is truly owner's pride & neighbor’s envy. I hope it will create huge waves in the circles of the learned so that the knowledge presented will percolate into every nook & corner of every community, educating the masses about the field of Homeopathy in Veterinary diseases.

I also wish Dr Muhammad K S all success in his future endeavors. Being a doctor, manufacturer & distributor of Homoeopathic medicines, I feel both honored & glad that the privilege of writing the foreword has been extended to me.

Let each of us remember the glorious past of Homeopathy & hope for an equally bright future for it.

Thank you & warm regards.

Dr. Sophia Zacharias
CEO & Managing Partner
St. George's Homoeopathy

FOREWORD

It is with immense pride and anticipation that I introduce the second edition of "POULTRY HOMEOPATHY - Advancing Homeopathic Research in Poultry Healthcare." Authored by the esteemed Dr. Muhammed KS, this edition builds upon the success of the first and continues to elevate the discourse in the field of poultry health.

Dr. Muhammed KS, a seasoned healthcare professional, has consistently demonstrated an unwavering commitment to pushing the boundaries of homeopathic research. With a wealth of experience and a diverse background in healthcare, Dr. Muhammed brings a unique perspective to the intersection of homeopathy and poultry health.

This edition delves even deeper into the nuances of homeopathic solutions for poultry, providing valuable insights into managing various health challenges faced by avian species. Dr. Muhammed's dedication to advancing homeopathic research in poultry healthcare is evident throughout the pages of this comprehensive and meticulously researched work.

The inclusion of the latest updates, research methodologies, and practical applications makes this edition an indispensable resource for practitioners, researchers, and anyone passionate about the well-being of poultry through homeopathic interventions.

As colleagues (Team Dezmons) in the homeopathic community, we commend Dr. Muhammed KS for his tireless efforts in advancing homeopathic research, and we are confident that this second edition will serve as a beacon for further exploration and innovation in the realm of poultry health.

ACKNOWLEDGMENTS

I extend my heartfelt appreciation to all those who have directly or indirectly contributed to the development of this book:

1. Dr. Hadiya, whose editorial expertise greatly enhanced the quality of the content.

2. Dr. Wakchaure Sanket Vinayak, BVSc, MVSc, for providing valuable updates on veterinary technical data.

3. Mrs. Devi Kumari. S, MA B.Ed. (English) and Dr. Mansoor Ali, BHMS for meticulously proof reading the primary text.

4. A special note of thanks to Dr. Shanu Salim MD Dr. Sudhi TK, BHMS, BSc Zoology, for their invaluable guidance that played a pivotal role in completing this book.

5. My sincere gratitude goes to Rose Publications and My Health Guide Publication for their unwavering support in bringing this book to publication.

POULTRY HOMEOPATHY

"Advancing Homeopathic Research in Poultry Healthcare"

2nd Edition

TABLE OF CONTENTS

POULTRY HOMEOPATHY

"Advancing Homeopathic Research in Poultry Healthcare"

2nd Edition

SECTION-1

INTRODUCTION

In recent times, the field of homeopathy has emerged as a compelling avenue for research and development. Homeopaths need not solely rely on governmental authorities for driving progress in this field. Instead, it is incumbent upon us to proactively enhance the quality and quantity of our research efforts to elevate the efficacy of homeopathic medicine.

The contemporary landscape is marked by the rise of private organizations and institutions that actively promote homeopathy. It is imperative that we harness these opportunities. Every dedicated homeopath should embark on individual research endeavors in their areas of interest, collectively contributing to the evolution of homeopathic medicine. Homeopathy, as a system of healing, boasts a rich history. However, it is crucial to acknowledge that progress has remained relatively stagnant over the past century. Far too often, we find ourselves reiterating the same concepts and principles established by our esteemed masters.

Our revered pioneers have bequeathed us an invaluable tool for human healthcare. Now, it is our responsibility to adapt this system to the demands of modern technology and transform it into a medical approach that anticipates the needs of the future.

The poultry industry presents a promising frontier for homeopathic research. Here, we can seamlessly apply rigorous scientific methodologies for drug validation. Poultry, as experimental subjects, offer an exceptional advantage. The life span of broiler birds is a mere 42 days, during which they are susceptible to a wide array of diseases.

This presents a unique opportunity to demonstrate the effectiveness of homeopathic treatments within a relatively short timeframe. Such proving of homeopathic remedies in poultry not only contributes to the creation of a valuable primary database for drug development but also paves the way for more extensive studies in the future.

HOMEOPATHIC SYSTEM OF MEDICINE

Homeopathy: A Holistic Approach to Health

Homeopathy is an alternative form of medical science dedicated to the comprehensive healthcare management of living beings. It has evolved to encompass practices that are designed not only to treat illness but also to maintain and restore complete health. The Homeopathic approach to disease management includes critical components such as diagnosis, prognosis, prevention, and treatment.

The inception of Homeopathy dates back to 1796 when it was introduced by Dr. Samuel Hahnemann, a German physician. It was under his guidance that the term 'Allopathy' was coined in 1810. The very name 'Homeopathy' finds its roots in the Greek words 'Homoeos,' meaning 'similar,' and 'pathos,' which signifies 'suffering disease.' The fundamental principle of Homeopathy is founded upon 'Similia, Similibus Curentur,' meaning 'like cures like.' Dr. Hahnemann was not merely the inventor of this system; he was also a visionary who meticulously developed every facet of Homeopathy, drawing upon his own experimental and pharmacological skills.

Dr. Samuel Hahnemann's significant contributions to the Homeopathic system of medicine include:

- **Basic Principles:** He introduced the fundamental principle of Homeopathy, 'Similia, Similibus Curentur,' which forms the cornerstone of this system.

- **Homeopathic Pharmaceutics:** Dr. Hahnemann devised precise methods for the preparation of homeopathic remedies, which are integral to the practice.
- **Drug Index:** His extensive work in Materia Medica Pura, spanning from Part-1 to Part-4, provided a comprehensive guide to the properties and uses of various homeopathic medicines.
- **Homeopathic Philosophy:** The 'Organon of Medicines,' presented in six parts, delves into the underlying philosophy and principles that govern the practice of Homeopathy.
- **Experimental Pharmacological Notes:**
  In his works like 'Chronic Disease and Peculiar Nature of the Homeopathic Cure' (Part-1 to 4), Dr. Hahnemann ventured into experimental pharmacology, further enhancing the understanding of the Homeopathic system and its effectiveness.
- **Miasmatic Theory:** Hahnemann introduced the concept of miasms, which are underlying disease tendencies inherited from ancestors. Understanding and addressing these miasms became an essential aspect of homeopathic treatment. miasmatic theory and modern genetic variability share some common ground in recognizing the importance of individualized approaches to health, they differ in their theoretical underpinnings, diagnostic tools, clinical applications, and levels of scientific validation. Miasmatic theory is specific to homeopathy, whereas genetic variability is a widely accepted concept within the broader field of genetics and modern medicine.

- **Impact on Modern Healthcare:**
  While homeopathy has evolved since Hahnemann's time, his contributions laid the groundwork for exploring alternative approaches to healing. The emphasis on individualized care and the minimization of side effects align with contemporary trends in patient-centered healthcare.

These contributions collectively demonstrate the depth of knowledge, dedication, and innovation that Dr. Samuel Hahnemann brought to the field of Homeopathy, making it a remarkable and enduring system of medicine.

Future Homeopathy Medicine: Unlocking New Frontiers in Holistic Healing: As we step into the future, homeopathy is poised to explore new horizons in the realm of holistic medicine. With advancements in scientific understanding and cutting-edge technologies, the development of homeopathic medicines is expected to become more precise and tailored to individual needs.

- Personalized Remedies: Future homeopathic medicines may leverage advanced diagnostic tools and genetic insights to tailor remedies more precisely. Individualized treatment plans based on genetic predispositions and unique symptomatology could enhance therapeutic outcomes.
- Integration with Conventional Medicine:
  As research continues to bridge the gap between conventional and alternative medicine, the integration of homeopathy into mainstream healthcare may become more seamless. Collaborative efforts could lead to comprehensive

treatment approaches that address diverse aspects of health.

- Technological Innovations: The use of advanced technologies, such as artificial intelligence and machine learning, may play a role in materia medica analysis and remedy selection. These innovations could streamline the process of finding the most effective homeopathic solutions for various health conditions.
- Evidence-Based Practice: Ongoing research endeavors seek to provide a more robust scientific foundation for homeopathy. Future developments may bring forth a wealth of empirical evidence supporting the efficacy of homeopathic treatments, contributing to increased acceptance within the broader medical community.
- Expanded Understanding of Vital Force: As our understanding of the vital force – a central concept in homeopathy – deepens, future medicines may aim to target and modulate this force more effectively. Exploring the interface between mind, body, and energy could open up new avenues for healing.
- Sustainable and Eco-Friendly Practices: With a growing emphasis on sustainability, future homeopathic medicine production may prioritize environmentally friendly practices. From sourcing raw materials to manufacturing processes, a commitment to eco-consciousness could define the industry.

While the future of homeopathy holds exciting possibilities, it's essential to balance innovation with the foundational principles laid down by pioneers like Dr. Samuel

Hahnemann. The holistic, patient-centered approach that has been at the core of homeopathy is likely to remain a guiding principle as the field continues to evolve.

SOURCES OF HOMEOPATHIC MEDICINES

Throughout history, plants have served as one of the most ancient and foundational sources of medicinal remedies. Many of the earliest medications were derived from plants and were informed by the practices of traditional and folk medicine. In the year 1869, a significant milestone was reached with the discovery of the first synthetic drug, chloral hydrate. As we progressed into the early 20th century, the scope of homeopathic medicines expanded to include substances from animal and mineral origins. Examples of these include adrenaline, liver extracts, iron, calcium, and more.

Dr. Samuel Hahnemann, the founder of Homeopathy, meticulously developed this system through extensive experiments and clinical trials. He tested over 4000 substances from various sources, laying the foundation for the Homeopathic Materia Medica. A substantial portion of homeopathic drugs is derived from plant sources.

These sources of homeopathic medicines can be broadly categorized as follows:

Plant Sources: These encompass the entire spectrum of plant materials, from roots, stems, leaves, fruits, seeds, barks, and wood to juices and constituents like alkaloids, glycosides, and resinoids.

Animal Sources: Homeopathic medicines derived from animals may involve whole animals, specific body parts or organs, excretions, biological materials, and even venoms.

Mineral Sources: This category includes acids (both organic and inorganic), elements, and various chemical compounds.

Nosodes (Bio-therapeutics): Introduced in 1833 by Dr. Hering, nosodes are developed from isopathic remedies. Dr. Hering conducted extensive experiments with isopathic remedies on humans, contributing to the innovative concept of bio-therapeutics in Homeopathy.

Sarcodes: These remedies are prepared from healthy organs, secretions, and tissues and are used to aid in the restoration of specific organ health.

Imponderabilia: Imponderabilia preparations are derived from natural and artificial physical energy sources.

Tautopathic: These remedies are sourced from synthetic substances.

Allersodes: Homeopathically potentized remedies created from various antigens, which are used as adjuvants in allergen immunotherapy.

Isodes: Medicines that are derived from causative agents of diseases.

Dr. Samuel Hahnemann outlined a unique and meticulous technical procedure for preparing homeopathic drugs from these diverse sources. The process, described in Organon of Medicine (Aphorisms 264 to 271),

Consists of two main steps:

1. **Mother Tincture or Solution Preparation:** This is the initial stage of creating homeopathic remedies.

2. **Potentization:** A unique and fundamental process in homeopathy, this involves quantified dilution and vigorous shaking, which systematically enhances the efficacy of the medicinal properties.

In the practice of Homeopathy, there are three key distinctions:

In the intricate realm of Homeopathy, practitioners navigate three pivotal distinctions that form the backbone of this holistic healing system:

1. **Drug:** Any therapeutic agent that can induce changes in an organism's physiological or pathological state when administered.
2. **Medicine:** A homeopathic drug that has been potentized and tested on healthy individuals, producing specific abnormal signs and symptoms.
3. **Remedy:** A specific medicine prescribed for particular health disorders, adhering to the core principle of Homeopathy.The term "potentization" is a defining feature of Homeopathy, contributing to the preparation of medicines from various sources. Proper selection of remedies, informed by the law of similars and the principles of Homeopathy, assures the efficacy, safety, and curative potential of these remedies for patients.

In embracing the threefold distinctions of Drug, Medicine, and Remedy, Homeopathy unveils a unique and profound approach to healing. The term "potentization" stands as a beacon, illuminating the preparation of medicines sourced from nature's vast repertoire. Through the unwavering adherence to the law of similars and Homeopathic principles, practitioners assure patients of remedies that transcend mere treatment—offering efficacy, safety, and the promise of true healing.

Drug Development Process:

Embarking on the journey of drug development in Homeopathy is a meticulous and multifaceted process, encompassing several indispensable steps. Each stage contributes to the overarching goal of ensuring the safety, efficacy, and quality of the eventual drug. This intricate process unfolds with a strategic approach, acknowledging the diverse nature of drug sources and adhering to stringent guidelines. From source identification to dosage determination, every phase is carefully orchestrated to uphold the integrity and authenticity of the drug. Let's delve into the essential stages that shape the trajectory of Homeopathic drug development. The process of developing a new drug involves several key steps to ensure its safety, efficacy, and quality.

1. **Source Identification:** Identifying the source of the drug is the first crucial step. Depending on the nature and origin of the substance, specific source identification rules need to be followed to maintain the quality and authenticity of the drug.
2. **Collection of Drug Substance:** The collection of the drug substance should adhere to precise guidelines, tailored to the nature and characteristics

of the sources. These rules ensure the integrity and quality of the collected material.

3. **Method of Preparation:** The method of preparing the drug varies depending on the nature of the substance. It is essential to follow a systematic and standardized approach to ensure the reproducibility and consistency of the drug.
4. **Quality Control:** Quality control measures, as defined by the Homeopathic Pharmacopoeia of India (HPI) or relevant guidelines, must be rigorously implemented to assess and maintain the quality of the drug.
5. **Drug Proving:** Before a drug is administered to patients, it must undergo proving, which includes human and animal trials. This step aims to understand the effects and safety of the drug, helping to establish its suitability for therapeutic use.
6. **Drug Dosage:** Determining the appropriate dosage is a critical aspect of drug development. This involves defining the minimum and maximum doses:
   - **Minimum Dose:** The concept of the minimum dose in Homeopathy revolves around administering the smallest concentration of the drug that can achieve maximum efficacy without inducing adverse effects. This delicate balance seeks to harness the curative potential of the remedy while minimizing any unwanted reactions. Identifying the minimum effective dose is pivotal for optimizing therapeutic benefits and aligns with the fundamental Homeopathic principle of "like cures like."

- **Maximum Dose:** Conversely, the maximum dose represents the highest concentration of the drug that can be safely administered to an individual at a given time without resulting in adverse effects. Striking a delicate equilibrium between therapeutic efficacy and safety, the determination of the maximum dose is guided by meticulous observation and adherence to Homeopathic principles. This ensures that the remedy's healing potential is harnessed while mitigating any risk of harm.

Each of these steps in the drug development process plays a vital role in ensuring that the resulting drug is of high quality, safe for use, and effective in treating the intended health conditions. The culmination of a Homeopathic drug's journey from inception to therapeutic fruition reflects a commitment to excellence and precision. The rigor of source identification, meticulous collection, standardized preparation methods, and stringent quality control measures collectively weave the fabric of a drug's integrity. The pivotal phase of drug proving, encompassing human and animal trials, underscores the commitment to understanding the drug's effects and safety profile. As the dosage parameters are meticulously defined – from the minimum dose optimizing therapeutic benefits to the maximum safe concentration – the drug development process ensures a holistic approach to delivering high-quality, safe, and efficacious solutions for diverse health conditions. Each step serves as a testament to the unwavering dedication to the principles of Homeopathy in crafting remedies that stand as beacons of healing excellence.

HISTORY AND EVOLUTION OF VETERINARY HOMEOPATHY

Veterinary homeopathy is a holistic approach to animal health that involves the use of highly diluted substances to stimulate the body's inherent healing mechanisms. Similar to homeopathy for humans, veterinary homeopathy operates on the principles of "like cures like" and individualization of treatment.

Veterinary Homeopathy is not a recent concept; its roots trace back to the early 18th century when the pioneering figure, Dr. Samuel Hahnemann (1755-1843), discussed the application of homeopathy in animals. During a lecture at the University of Leipzig, one of Germany's oldest academic institutions, he emphasized that **the principles and application of homeopathy in animals closely mirrored those in humans.** This marked the nascent stage of Veterinary Homeopathy.

The evolution of this field took significant strides when individuals like Boenninghausen and Lux expanded upon Dr. Hahnemann's work. Boenninghausen introduced essential homeopathic treatment protocols for animals, heralding a momentous leap in the practice of Veterinary Homeopathy.

In the 19th century, Mr. George Macleod (1912-1995) emerged as a prominent Veterinary Homeopath in the United Kingdom. He played a pivotal role in advancing the field and was the founder of the British Association of Homeopathic Veterinary Surgeons.

On an international scale, the International Association for Veterinary Homeopathy (IAVH) was established in Luxembourg in 1986. The association held its first Congress in Oxford (UK) in 1987. Over the years, the IAVH has been instrumental in guiding teaching programs globally and in setting standards for examinations leading to the qualification of Cert. IAVH.

In more recent times, a postgraduate certified course in veterinary homeopathy has been made available in New Zealand at the College of Natural Health and Homeopathy. This institution has been a significant provider of homeopathic education since 1989, with a strong presence in Auckland and Tauranga.

In India, the first veterinary homeopathic courses were introduced in 2016, specifically at the Kerala Veterinary and Animal Science University (KVASU) located in Thrissur, Mannuthy. These courses offer a Post Graduate Certificate in Veterinary Homeopathy (PGCVH) designed for veterinary doctors. Additionally, private organizations now provide personalized training for professionals interested in Veterinary Homeopathy. The field of Veterinary Homeopathy has advanced considerably, and the availability of Homeopathic Veterinary Solutions Software is a testament to the progress made in this specialized branch of homeopathic practice.

In recent times, homeopathy has gained recognition and acceptance as an effective and holistic approach in the management of various health issues across different kinds of livestock. This shift toward using homeopathy in livestock reflects a growing awareness of sustainable and natural alternatives to conventional medical practices.

Rise of Homeopathy in Livestock Management:

Over the past few years, there has been a notable increase in the use of homeopathy for the health and well-being of livestock, including poultry, cattle, swine, and other animals. This shift is driven by several factors:

Reducing Dependency on Conventional Medications:

Livestock owners and farmers are increasingly seeking alternatives to conventional medications, especially antibiotics. Homeopathy provides a non-invasive and natural approach, reducing the dependence on synthetic drugs.

Prevention and Prophylaxis:

Homeopathic remedies are often used for preventive measures, helping to boost the immune system and fortify the animals against common diseases. This emphasis on prophylaxis aligns with the goal of maintaining healthy livestock populations.

Addressing Concerns of Residue and Resistance: Homeopathic treatments do not leave residual substances in animal products, addressing concerns related to antibiotic residues. This is particularly important in the context of food safety and addressing the global issue of antibiotic resistance.

Research and Positive Outcomes:

Ongoing research and practical experiences are showcasing positive outcomes of using homeopathy in livestock. Farmers and veterinarians are reporting improvements in animal health, productivity, and overall well-being.

Challenges and Future Directions:

While the use of homeopathy in livestock is gaining popularity, challenges remain. Scientific validation, standardized protocols, and integration into mainstream veterinary practices are areas that require further attention. Continued collaboration between homeopathic practitioners, veterinarians, and researchers is crucial for advancing the understanding and effectiveness of homeopathic approaches in diverse livestock settings.

In conclusion, the current trend toward using homeopathy in all kinds of livestock underscores a paradigm shift in animal healthcare, emphasizing natural, holistic, and sustainable practices for the benefit of both animals and consumers.

Homeopathy in Animal Health:

Homeopathy in animal health involves a holistic understanding of the animal's constitution, behaviors, and symptoms. Rather than merely addressing isolated ailments, Homeopathy seeks to treat the entire being. Similar to its application in human health, Homeopathy in animal care revolves around individualized treatment plans. Remedies are chosen based on a detailed understanding of the animal's specific symptoms, temperament, and overall health profile. One of the distinctive features of Homeopathy is its focus on minimal doses. This not only contributes to the safety of the treatment but also minimizes the risk of side effects. Homeopathic remedies, derived from natural sources, are gentle yet potent, making them well-suited for various animals, including pets, livestock, and wildlife. By strengthening the animal's overall vitality and immune system, Homeopathic treatments can play a role in preventing diseases and supporting the animal's well-being throughout its life.

Integration with Conventional Veterinary Care:

Homeopathy can complement conventional veterinary care, offering an integrative approach to animal health. Collaborative efforts between Homeopathic practitioners and conventional veterinarians can provide a more comprehensive and synergistic approach to managing a range of health conditions in animals.

In essence, Homeopathy in animal health reflects a commitment to the holistic and individualized care of our animal companions. By embracing the principles of Homeopathy, animals can experience gentle yet effective healing, promoting their overall health and vitality.

Exploring the Global Landscape of Veterinary Homeopathy: Countries, Practices, and Regulations

Here are some countries where veterinary homeopathy is generally recognized and practiced:

1. India: Veterinary homeopathy is widely practiced, and there are homeopathic remedies specifically formulated for animals.
2. Germany: Veterinary homeopathy is accepted and practiced alongside conventional veterinary medicine.
3. United Kingdom: Veterinary homeopathy is practiced, and there are veterinarians who integrate homeopathic treatments into their practice.
4. France: Veterinary homeopathy is used in France, and there are homeopathic veterinary practitioners.

5. United States: Veterinary homeopathy is practiced, and some veterinarians offer homeopathic treatments for animals.
6. Brazil: Veterinary homeopathy is recognized, and there are homeopathic veterinary practitioners.
7. Australia: Veterinary homeopathy is practiced, and there are veterinarians who use homeopathic remedies for animals.
8. Canada: Veterinary homeopathy is available, and some veterinarians incorporate homeopathic treatments.

It's important to consider that regulations and acceptance can vary within countries, and the level of integration into mainstream veterinary practices may differ. Additionally, regulations can change, so it's advisable to check with relevant veterinary authorities or professional organizations for the latest information on rules and regulations regarding veterinary homeopathy in a specific country.

Reputable Institutions Offering Veterinary Homeopathy Courses Worldwide"

1. College of Veterinary and Animal Sciences.
   Mannuthy, Thrissur, Kerala. Courses Details: Post graduate certificate in Veterinary Homoeopathy (PGCVH).
2. College of Veterinary and Animal Sciences.
   Pookode, Vythiri, Kerala. Courses Details: Post graduate certificate in Veterinary Homoeopathy (PGCVH).
3. The Royal Animal Health University (RAHU) – United Kingdom. Courses Details: Veterinary

homeopathy. Website: The Royal Animal Health University.

4. The British Institute of Homeopathy - United Kingdom, Provides courses in classical homeopathy for both humans and animals.
   Website: British Institute of Homeopathy.
5. Hahnemann College of Homeopathy - United States Provides courses in classical homeopathy for both humans and animals.
   Website: Hahnemann College of Homeopathy
6. The National Academy of Homeopathy - United States Offers courses in classical homeopathy.
   Website: National Academy of Homeopathy
7. The Australasian College of Hahnemannian Homoeopathy (ACHH) – Australia
   Provides courses in homeopathy, including veterinary applications.
   Website: Australasian College of Hahnemannian Homoeopathy
8. The Allen College of Homeopathy - United Kingdom. Offers courses in classical homeopathy.
   Website: Allen College of Homeopathy
9. Hogrefe Academy – Germany
   Provides courses in veterinary homeopathy.
   Website: Hogrefe Academy
10. Centro de Formación de Terapeutas Naturales – Spain Offers courses in homeopathy with veterinary applications. Website: Centro de Formación de Terapeutas Naturales

SCOPE OF HOMEOPATHIC RESEARCH IN POULTRY

Use of Homeopathic medicines for animals known as Veterinary Homeopathy.

Scope of Homeopathic Research in Poultry

The use of homeopathic medicines for animals, often referred to as Veterinary Homeopathy, holds significant potential, particularly in the context of organic farming. The poultry industry, in particular, has been actively promoting homeopathic therapies. In poultry, there are four key treatment protocols in Veterinary Homeopathy:

1. **Constitutional Therapies:** These involve the use of constitutional medicines tailored to the individual bird's symptoms and needs, emphasizing the principle of individualization.
2. **Miasmatic Treatment**: Miasmatic remedies are employed to address underlying miasmatic conditions in poultry.
3. **Therapeutic Management:** This approach is based on the pharmacological actions of homeopathic medicines, where specific remedies are chosen for their therapeutic effects.
4. **Isopathic Protocols:** This encompasses various immune-therapies, bio-therapies using substances from living organisms, and organopathy, which involves specific remedies for individual organs.

In the field of homeopathy, the process of drug development and medicinal experimentation adheres to stringent guidelines. In homeopathy, drug development is known as

"Drug Proving," which is the systematic process of acquiring knowledge about substances used for the treatment of natural diseases. (Aphorism-105, Homeopathic Pharmacopoeia of India, 2nd Edition, Mandal and Madal, 2004).

Two fundamental methodologies are employed in the Homeopathic System of Medicines for drug proving:

A. Animal Proving

B. Human Proving

Three critical aspects to consider during the drug proving process are:

1. Drug Quality: Ensuring the quality and purity of the substance being tested.
2. Prover: Engaging healthy and well-qualified individuals for proving.
3. Environment: Providing a controlled and normal environment for conducting the proving.

Ethical Guidelines for the Use of Animals in Research

When conducting scientific research and testing involving animals, ethical considerations are of utmost importance. In 1959, W.M. Russel and R.L. Burch introduced the "3R Principle" as a fundamental guideline for the ethical use of animals in research:

- **Replace:** Prioritize efforts to seek alternatives to animal testing whenever possible.
- **Reduce:** Modify experimental protocols to minimize the number of animals required for research.

- **Refinement:** Focus on measures that minimize the severity of suffering, pain, and stress experienced by the animals involved in research.

By adhering to these ethical guidelines, researchers can balance the pursuit of scientific knowledge with the humane treatment of animals, ensuring the highest standards of ethical conduct in research and testing.

ROUTES OF DRUG ADMINISTRATION AND DRUG DOSAGE FORMS

While the most common method of administering homeopathic medicines is orally, Homeopathy offers various routes of drug administration. The choice of administration route depends on factors such as the patient's condition, the nature of the medicine, and individual preferences, including those of the physician. Homeopathic drug administration routes are broadly categorized into,

1. **Systemic Routes**
   a. **Oral:** The most prevalent method, where medicines are taken by mouth.
   b. **Sub-lingual (Buccal)**: Involves placing the medicine under the tongue for absorption through the mucous membranes.
   c. **Cutaneous (Epidermic and Enepidermic):** Application on the skin, which can be further divided into external (on the skin surface) and internal (absorbed through the skin).
   d. **Inhalation:** Administered through olfaction, either by inhaling through the nose or mouth.
   e. **Nasal, Ear, and Eyes:** Medicines can be administered through the nasal passage, ears, or eyes when required.

2. **Local Routes**
   a. **Topical (External Application):** Medicine is applied externally to the affected area or skin surface.

b. **Sub-lingual (Buccal):** Similar to systemic use, it can also be administered locally when focusing on specific oral or buccal conditions.
c. **Cutaneous (Epidermic and Enepidermic):** Like systemic use, medicines can be applied externally on the skin for localized effects.
d. **Inhalation:** Inhalation through the nose or mouth can be used for targeted local treatment.
e. **Nasal:** Specific application through the nasal passages can be employed for localized conditions.

Homeopathic Drug Dosage Forms

Homeopathic medicines are available in various dosage forms, ensuring that they are convenient and effective for patients. These forms cater to different patient needs and preferences:

1. **Solid Dosage Forms**: These include homeopathic pills, tablets, and granules, designed for oral consumption. They are easy to handle and provide a precise dosage.
2. **Liquid Dosage Forms**: Liquid homeopathic medicines can be taken orally, and they include tinctures, solutions, and syrups. These forms offer flexibility in dosing and are suitable for patients who prefer liquid medication.
3. **Semisolid Dosage Forms:** Semisolid forms like ointments and creams are designed for topical application. They are effective for treating skin conditions and external ailments.

The diversity of drug administration routes and dosage forms in Homeopathy ensures that patients can receive their treatment in a manner that best suits their specific needs and the nature of their condition.

THE ROLE OF HOMEOPATHY IN POULTRY FARMING

Homeopathy presents a promising future in poultry farming, offering a valuable tool for farmers and contributing to the welfare of the poultry industry. Poultry is the second most widely consumed meat globally, and Homeopathy can play a pivotal role in enhancing the health of poultry birds and ensuring the safety of poultry meat for consumers. The significance of Homeopathy in poultry farming aligns with the broader concept of organic farming, which seeks to improve health and safety, foster economic and social benefits, and reduce environmental impact.

Why Homeopathy in Poultry Farming?

In recent years, the integration of homeopathy into poultry farming practices has gained attention as a holistic and sustainable approach to enhance the health and well-being of poultry. Homeopathy, a system of alternative medicine founded on the principle of "like cures like," focuses on stimulating the body's innate healing mechanisms. Applied to poultry farming, homeopathy offers a natural and preventive method that aligns with the principles of organic and sustainable agriculture. This approach considers the interconnectedness of environmental factors, animal welfare, and overall farm health.

- **Antibiotic Resistance & Ban:** With the growing concern of antibiotic resistance, Homeopathy provides a viable alternative for disease management in poultry, especially in light of antibiotic bans and regulations. The Key Aspects of

Antibiotic Resistance & Homeopathic Alternatives are follows

1. Global Antibiotic Resistance Crisis.
2. Regulations and Antibiotic Bans.
3. Homeopathy as a Sustainable Alternative.
4. Antibiotic-Free Livestock
5. Reduced Environmental Impact

- **Dominance in Anti-Viral Management:** Homeopathy has shown superiority in managing viral diseases in poultry. The significance of the Homeopathy in its role in anti-viral management has become increasingly evident, highlighting the potential for improved outcomes and reduced reliance on conventional pharmaceutical interventions.
- **Superiority in Prophylaxis Care**: Homeopathic treatments are effective in prophylactic care, contributing to disease prevention. Homeopathy emerges as a superior choice in the realm of prophylaxis care, showcasing its efficacy in preventing diseases and fostering a robust defense mechanism.
- **No Side Effects and Zero Harm:** Homeopathic remedies are well-known for their safety, as they have no side effects and pose no harm to poultry birds.
- **Cost-Effective:** Homeopathic treatments are often more cost-effective than traditional pharmaceutical options.

- **Organic Farming:** Homeopathy aligns with the principles of organic farming, supporting sustainable and chemical-free poultry practices. Organic farming holds several potential benefits for future healthcare, both in terms of environmental sustainability and potential impacts on human health. Organic livestock farming typically prohibits the routine use of antibiotics for growth promotion. This can help reduce the development of antibiotic-resistant bacteria, which is a significant concern for human health.

In conclusion, the incorporation of homeopathy into poultry farming reflects a broader shift toward sustainable and natural farming practices. By emphasizing preventive healthcare, reducing dependency on antibiotics, and adopting a holistic approach to poultry well-being, homeopathy aligns with the goals of modern, environmentally conscious agriculture. While challenges and skepticism may exist, ongoing research and successful case studies contribute to the growing acceptance of homeopathy as a valuable tool in promoting the health and productivity of poultry farms. As the agricultural landscape evolves, homeopathy stands as a promising avenue for fostering resilient and sustainable poultry farming systems.

Advantages of Poultry Birds for Ethical Research

Poultry birds stand as invaluable subjects for ethical research in the realms of homeopathy and veterinary science, offering a multitude of advantages that contribute to the advancement of knowledge and the development of ethical practices. These avian subjects present unique characteristics and suitability for various types of trials, comparative studies, and investigations into the efficacy and safety of homeopathic treatments.

Poultry birds offer several advantages for ethical research in the field of homeopathy and veterinary science:

- **Easily Accessible:** Poultry birds are readily available and accessible as research subjects.
- **Natural Disease Occurrence:** Poultry birds naturally contract various diseases within a short span of 42 days, making them ideal for conducting trials without artificially creating diseases.
- **Various Types of Trials:** Poultry birds are suitable for diverse trials, including treatment trials, prevention trials, and synchronized trials.
- **Comparative Studies:** Comparative studies are feasible, allowing for assessments of homeopathic remedies against competitor products such as antibiotics, vaccines, and other treatment methods.
- **Challenge Studies:** Poultry birds are suitable for challenge studies to ensure the therapeutic efficacy of homeopathic treatments.
- **Efficacy Parameters:** Researchers can analyze various efficacy parameters in poultry birds, including blood, blood serum, biochemical markers, blood smears, and organ analysis.
- **Toxicological Studies:** Poultry birds can be used for toxicological studies to assess the safety and potential toxicity of treatments.
- **Laboratory and Field Experiments:** Both laboratory and field experiments can be conducted with poultry birds.

- **Similar Health Conditions to Humans:** Poultry birds often experience health conditions similar to those in humans, making them a relevant model for homeopathic research.
- **Biological Similarity:** Approximately 60% of chicken genes are similar to human genes, allowing for treatments that are comparable to human protocols.
- **Physiological Actions:** Poultry birds help evaluate the physiological actions of homeopathic drugs.
- **Longitudinal Studies:** Researchers can conduct whole lifespan studies and multi-generational cross studies.
- **Challenge Studies (Diet and Environment):** Researchers can control diet and environmental conditions in challenge studies.
- **Safety and Toxicity Testing:** Poultry birds provide a solution for testing the safety and toxicity of homeopathic treatments.
- **Experimental Pharmacology:** Poultry birds are suitable for experimental pharmacology studies, contributing to the understanding of drug actions.
- **Pre-Clinical Research:** They can be used for pre-clinical research tests to assess the potential of homeopathic medicines.
- **Adverse Drug Reactions:** Poultry birds offer insights into adverse drug reactions, enhancing safety assessments.

The advantages presented by poultry birds in ethical research are extensive and diverse, making them pivotal contributors to the advancement of homeopathy and veterinary science. Their accessibility, biological similarities, and suitability for various types of studies position poultry birds as ethical and reliable subjects, offering valuable insights into the safety, efficacy, and potential applications of homeopathic treatments. As ethical considerations become increasingly significant in research practices, poultry birds remain at the forefront, playing a vital role in shaping the future of homeopathic and veterinary science research.

TRIAL PARAMETERS IN POULTRY RESEARCH

Poultry research involves a range of trial parameters to assess the health, performance, and well-being of poultry birds. These parameters are broadly categorized as basic (observatory) parameters and specific (investigatory) parameters, play a pivotal role in understanding and optimizing poultry production practices.

1. Basic (Observatory) Parameters:

- **Feed Intake (FI)**
  Monitoring the quantity of feed consumed by poultry birds, a crucial metric influencing overall health and productivity.

- **Weight (WT)**
  Measuring the body weight of birds, a fundamental parameter reflecting growth and development.

- **FCR (Feed Conversion Ratio)**
  Calculating the efficiency of feed conversion, representing the ratio of feed intake to body weight and providing insights into resource utilization.

- **Mortality**
  Tracking bird deaths, a critical indicator of the health and welfare of the poultry flock.

- **Meat Yield**
  Assessing the quantity and quality of meat produced, essential for evaluating the economic viability of poultry farming.

- **Production Cost:**
  Evaluating the overall cost associated with poultry production, aiding in financial management and decision-making.

- **EEF (European Efficiency Factor)**
  A comprehensive factor that standardizes technical results by considering feed conversion, mortality, and daily gain, providing a holistic view of efficiency.

  The formula is: (Average grams gained per day X % survival rate) / Feed Conversion Ratio X 10.

2. Specific (Investigatory) Parameters:

- **Blood Analysis:** Comprehensive blood tests that include Total Blood Cell Count, Red Blood Cell Count (RBC), Hemoglobin Percentage (Hb%), White Blood Cell Count (WBC), Packed Cell Volume (PCV), Mean Corpuscular Volume (MCV), Hematocrit (HCT), and Platelet count.
- **Blood Biochemical Parameters:** Analyzing blood for glucose levels, cholesterol levels, HDL (High-Density Lipoprotein) cholesterol, LDL (Low-Density Lipoprotein) cholesterol, VLDL (Very Low-Density Lipoprotein) cholesterol, as well as mineral levels such as calcium (Ca), phosphorus (Phosphorous), zinc (Zn), manganese, copper, iron, iodine, and selenium. Vitamin levels are also examined.
- **Blood Serum Analysis:** Assessing the serum for markers such as the Erythrocyte Sedimentation Rate (ESR) and specific titers related to diseases like MG

(Mycoplasma gallisepticum), IB (Infectious Bronchitis), IBD (Infectious Bursal Disease), ND (Newcastle Disease).

- **Blood Smear Analysis:** Determining the H: L Ratio (Heterophil to Lymphocyte ratio) to evaluate immune responses.
- **Samples Analysis:** Examining immune organs (Thymus, Bursa, Spleen, and Liver), as well as the weight and histopathology of organs such as the kidney, gastrointestinal tract (GIT), bursa, gut, and respiratory organs.
- **Organ Examinations:** Scoring the health and condition of the gut and respiratory system, including gut score and respiratory score.

These trial parameters serve as a comprehensive toolkit for researchers and poultry farmers, offering invaluable insights into the intricate dynamics of poultry health and production. By judiciously examining basic and specific parameters, stakeholders can optimize management practices, enhance bird welfare, and achieve higher levels of efficiency in poultry farming. The integration of these parameters into research and farm management practices marks a crucial step towards the sustainable and ethical advancement of the poultry industry.

SECTION-2

POULTRY DISEASES & CLASSIFICATIONS

Disease incidence in the poultry sector can be attributed to various factors, with infectious agents playing a significant role. The occurrence of diseases not only threatens the health of poultry but also results in substantial economic losses for commercial poultry farmers. Effective disease classification is pivotal for accurate diagnosis and the proper management of poultry illnesses. Disease classification can be carried out based on different criteria, such as etiological, pathological, physiological, anatomical, epidemiological, and topographic factors.

In this context, disease classification is primarily organized chronologically, with the primary consideration given to the etiological factors. Subcategories are then classified according to pathological, physiological, and topographic criteria.

Scientific Classification of Chicken (Gallus Domesticus)

Domain: Eukaryote

Kingdom: Metazoan

Phylum: Chordata

Subphylum: Vertebrata

Class: Aves

Understanding and effectively managing poultry diseases is essential to safeguard the health and well-being of chickens (Gallus Domesticus) and to maintain the economic viability of poultry farming. Proper disease classification and research play a crucial role in achieving these goals.

Poultry diseases are a significant concern in the poultry industry, impacting bird health, productivity, and economic sustainability. Understanding the classifications of these diseases is crucial for effective management and preventive measures. Understanding the diverse nature of poultry diseases and their classifications is paramount for implementing targeted prevention and treatment strategies. Regular monitoring, biosecurity measures, and a holistic approach to bird health contribute to maintaining a sustainable and thriving poultry industry.

Types of Poultry Diseases

Poultry diseases encompass a diverse range of health issues affecting chickens and other avian species. These diseases are classified into various types based on their causative agents and presenting symptoms.

Infectious Diseases

I. Viral Diseases:

Viral diseases are a significant concern in poultry farming as they can cause high mortality rates, reduce productivity, and lead to economic losses.

- Avian Influenza: Also known as bird flu, it can lead to severe respiratory and systemic infections in poultry.
  Causative Agent: Influenza A virus, primarily subtypes H5 and H7.
  Transmission: Direct contact with infected birds, contaminated equipment, or through airborne particles.
  Symptoms: Respiratory distress, drop in egg production, swelling of the head, and sudden death.

Prevention and Control: Strict biosecurity measures, vaccination, Medicinal support and surveillance.

- Infectious Bronchitis: A highly contagious viral disease affecting the respiratory system of chickens.
  Causative Agent: Avian coronavirus.
  Transmission: Respiratory droplets and contact with contaminated surfaces.
  Symptoms: Respiratory distress, drop in egg production, kidney damage.
  Prevention and Control: Vaccination, biosecurity, Medicinal support and strict hygiene.

- Infectious Bursal Disease: Commonly known as Gumboro disease, it primarily targets the bursa of Fabricius.
  Causative Agent: Infectious bursal disease virus (IBDV).
  Transmission: Fecal-oral route, contaminated environment.
  Symptoms: Immunosuppression, swollen bursa, and increased mortality.
  Prevention and Control: Vaccination, Medicinal support and biosecurity.

- Newcastle Disease: A viral infection causing respiratory, nervous, and digestive symptoms.
  Causative Agent: Newcastle disease virus (NDV).
  Transmission: Inhalation of respiratory droplets, contact with contaminated feed or equipment.
  Symptoms: Respiratory signs, nervous signs, and drop in egg production.
  Prevention and Control: Vaccination, biosecurity, Medicinal support and proper hygiene.

- Marek’s Disease: A herpesvirus infection leading to tumors and immunosuppression.
  Causative Agent: Marek's disease virus (MDV).
  Transmission: Shedding of the virus in feather follicle dander.
  Symptoms: Tumors, paralysis, and poor growth.
  Prevention and Control: Vaccination, Medicinal support and good biosecurity practices.

- Chicken Anemia Disease: Causes anemia, poor growth, and increased mortality.
  Causative Agent: Chicken anemia virus (CAV).
  Transmission: Vertical transmission (from hen to chick), contaminated fomites.
  Symptoms: Anemia, weakness, and increased mortality in young chicks.
  Prevention and Control: Biosecurity, Medicinal support, culling infected birds, and minimizing vertical transmission.

- Egg Drops Syndrome: Known for a drop-in egg production and changes in egg quality.
  Causative Agent: Duck adenovirus type 1.
  Transmission: Fecal-oral route, contaminated water.
  Symptoms: Drop in egg production, soft-shelled and misshapen eggs.
  Prevention and Control: Biosecurity, Medicinal support and vaccination.

- Inclusion Body Hepatitis: Leads to liver damage and reduced growth.
  Causative Agent: Avihepatovirus, specifically fowl adenovirus serotype 8 (FAdV-8).

Transmission: Vertical Transmission. The virus is primarily transmitted vertically from infected hens to their progeny through the egg. It can also be horizontally transmitted among chicks.
Symptoms: Age Susceptibility: Typically affects chicks between 2 days and 3 weeks of age.
Prevention and Control: Vaccination, Medicinal support, Sanitation, Isolation, Culling.

- Infectious Laryngotracheitis (ILT): Infectious Laryngotracheitis (ILT) is a highly contagious respiratory disease that affects chickens, primarily characterized by inflammation of the larynx and trachea. The disease is caused by Gallid herpesvirus type 1 (GaHV-1), also known as Infectious Laryngotracheitis Virus (ILTV).
  Causative Agent: Gallid herpesvirus type 1.
  Transmission: Respiratory droplets and direct contact.
  Symptoms: Respiratory distress, nasal discharge, and bloody mucus.
  Prevention and Control: Vaccination, Medicinal support, biosecurity, and quarantine.

- Fowl pox: Fowlpox is a viral disease that affects chickens and occasionally turkeys. It is caused by the Avipoxvirus, a member of the Poxviridae family. Fowlpox is characterized by the formation of wart-like lesions on the skin, mucous membranes, and occasionally the respiratory tract.
  Causative Agent: Avipoxvirus.
  Transmission: Mosquitoes and direct contact with infected birds or fomites.

Symptoms: Skin lesions, diphtheritic (wet) or cutaneous (dry) form.
Prevention and Control: Vaccination, Medicinal support and mosquito control.

- Chicken Astrovirus Infection: Chicken Astrovirus (CAstV) is a virus that infects chickens and belongs to the Astroviridae family. Astroviruses are known for causing gastroenteritis in various species, and in chickens, they have been associated with enteric diseases.
  Causative Agent: Chicken astrovirus.
  Transmission: Fecal-oral route.
  Symptoms: Enteritis, stunting, and retarded growth in chicks.
  Prevention and Control: Medicinal support Good hygiene practices and biosecurity.

II. **Bacterial Diseases:** Bacterial diseases are a significant concern in poultry farming, as they can cause various health issues and economic losses. Here are some common bacterial diseases in poultry:

- Avian Colibacillosis (E-COLI): A bacterial infection causing a range of symptoms, including diarrhea.
  Causative Agent: Escherichia coli (E. coli).
  Symptoms: Respiratory signs. Swollen joints and lameness.
  Peritonitis.
  Prevention and Control: Antibiotics, Vaccination, and sanitation.

- Necrotic Enteritis: Results in necrotic lesions in the intestine, also known as Clostridial Enteritis.

Causative Agent: Clostridium perfringens.
Symptoms: Sudden death, Diarrhea, Reduced growth.
Prevention and Control: Antibiotics, coccidiostats, and improved management practices.

- Fowl Cholera: Caused by Pasteurella multocida, it can lead to respiratory and systemic infections.
  Causative Agent: Pasteurella multocida.
  Symptoms: Sudden death, Swollen wattles and joints, Respiratory signs.
  Prevention and Control: Antibiotics, vaccination, and biosecurity.

- Avian Tuberculosis: Mycobacterium avium infection affecting various organs.
  Causative Agent: Mycobacterium avium.
  Symptoms: Weight loss, Swollen abdomen, Weakness.
  Prevention and Control: Antibiotics (although challenging), culling, and strict biosecurity.

III. **Mycoplasmosis:** Mycoplasmosis in poultry refers to infections caused by Mycoplasma species, **which are bacteria lacking a cell wall**. Mycoplasma infections are common in poultry and can lead to various diseases, with Mycoplasma gallisepticum (MG) and Mycoplasma synoviae (MS) being two significant pathogens.

- Mycoplasma Gallisepticum (Chronic Respiratory Disease): Affects the respiratory system.
  Causative Agent: Mycoplasma gallisepticum.
  Disease: Chronic Respiratory Disease (CRD).

Transmission: Airborne transmission, Vertical transmission from infected hens to chicks.
Symptoms: Respiratory signs (coughing, sneezing, nasal discharge), Swollen sinuses, Conjunctivitis, Reduced egg production and poor egg quality.
Prevention and Control: Antibiotics for infected flocks, Vaccination (live attenuated or inactivated vaccines), Biosecurity measures to prevent introduction and spread.

- Mycoplasma Synoviae (Infectious Synovitis): Causes joint infections.
  Causative Agent: Mycoplasma synoviae.
  Disease: Infectious Synovitis.
  Transmission: Vertical transmission, Direct contact with infected birds or contaminated fomites.
  Symptoms: Swollen joints (lameness), Respiratory signs, Decreased egg production and poor egg quality.
  Prevention and Control: Antibiotics for infected flocks, Vaccination (live or inactivated vaccines), Biosecurity measures to prevent introduction and spread.

- Mycoplasma meleagridis:
  Causative Agent: Mycoplasma meleagridis.
  Disease: Airsacculitis, Sinusitis, and Infertility in Turkeys.
  Symptoms: Respiratory signs, Swollen sinuses and airsacs, Reduced fertility in turkeys.
  Prevention and Control: Biosecurity measures.No commercially available vaccine; antibiotics may be used.

- Mycoplasma iowae:
  Causative Agent: Mycoplasma iowae.
  Disease: Mycoplasma Synoviae-Like Infection in Turkeys.
  Symptoms: Swollen joints, Respiratory signs, Poor growth.
  Prevention and Control: Biosecurity measures, No specific vaccine; antibiotics may be used.

IV. **Chlamydia:** Chlamydia refers to a group of bacteria belonging to the genus Chlamydia. In poultry, the most relevant species is Chlamydia psittaci, which can cause avian chlamydiosis, also known as psittacosis or ornithosis and Parrot Fever. Affects the respiratory system and may lead to flu-like symptoms.

Causative Agent: Chlamydia psittaci.
Transmission: Aerosol transmission (inhaling respiratory secretions, fecal dust, or contaminated feathers). Direct contact with infected birds or contaminated surfaces.
Host Range: Affects a wide range of bird species, including chickens, turkeys, pigeons, ducks, and psittacine birds (parrots).
Symptoms: Respiratory signs (nasal discharge, coughing, sneezing), Greenish diarrhea, Drop in egg production (in layer hens), General signs of illness such as lethargy and weight loss.
Zoonotic Potential: Humans can contract psittacosis from infected birds, causing flu-like symptoms.
Prevention and Control: Antibiotics (tetracyclines, macrolides) for infected birds. Strict biosecurity measures to prevent introduction and spread.

V. **Protozoal:** Protozoa are single-celled microscopic organisms that can be pathogenic to poultry. Protozoal infections in poultry are often associated with gastrointestinal or intestinal diseases.

- Coccidiosis: Coccidiosis is a common protozoal infection in poultry caused by various species of the Eimeria genus. These single-celled parasites can affect the intestinal tract of chickens, leading to a range of clinical signs and economic losses in poultry production.
  Causative Agent: Various species of Eimeria (e.g., Eimeria tenella, Eimeria acervulina).
  Transmission: Ingestion of sporulated oocysts from contaminated feed, water, or litter.
  Symptoms: Diarrhea (may contain blood), Reduced feed intake, Drooping wings and lethargy.
  Prevention and Control: Coccidiostats in feed, Proper sanitation, Rotational grazing, Vaccination in some cases.

- Histomoniasis (Blackhead Disease):
  Causative Agent: Histomonas meleagridis.
  Transmission: Fecal-oral route, often via the cecal worm Heterakis gallinarum.
  Symptoms: Cyanosis of the head (giving it a black appearance), Liver necrosis, Drooping wings and depression.
  Prevention and Control: Prevention of cecal worm infestation.
  Avoidance of contact with infected birds.

- Trichomoniasis (Canker):
  Causative Agent: Trichomonas gallinae.
  Transmission: Direct contact between birds, often through contaminated water.
  Prevention and Control: Yellowish cheesy growth in the mouth and throat. Reduced feed intake. Weight loss and drooping wings.
  Prevention and Control: Antiprotozoal medications (metronidazole), Hygiene measures to prevent contamination.

- Cryptosporidiosis:
  Causative Agent: Cryptosporidium spp.
  Transmission: Ingestion of oocysts from contaminated water or food.
  Symptoms: Diarrhea, Weight loss, Reduced growth.
  Prevention and Control: Proper sanitation, Clean water sources, Management practices to reduce stress.

- Hexamitiasis:
  Causative Agent: Hexamita meleagridis.
  Transmission: Fecal-oral route.
  Symptoms: Diarrhea, Weight loss, Reduced feed consumption.
  Prevention and Control: Antiprotozoal medications, Good management practices.

- Sarcocystosis:
  Causative Agent: Various Sarcocystis species.
  Transmission: Ingestion of sporocysts from contaminated feed, water, or intermediate hosts.
  Symptoms: Muscle inflammation and swelling, Reduced weight gain.

Prevention and Control: Proper cooking of feed ingredients.
Control of intermediate hosts.

VI. **Parasites:** Parasitic infestations are a common concern in poultry farming and can adversely affect the health and productivity of the birds. Various parasites, including internal and external types,

- Internal Parasites:
  Roundworms (Nematodes), Ascarids (Ascaridia galli), Heterakis gallinarum.
  Flatworms (Trematodes): Syngamus trachea (Gapeworm), Coccidia (Eimeria species).

- External Parasites:
  Mites: Dermanyssus gallinae (Red Mite) Transmission: Mites hide in cracks and crevices during the day and feed on birds at night. Symptoms: Anemia, reduced egg production, feather loss. Control: Acaricides, proper sanitation.
  Lice: Menopon gallinae (Biting Louse) and Goniodes spp. (Sucking Louse): Transmission: Direct contact between birds. Symptoms: Blood-feeding, irritation, Feather damage, irritation, reduced performance. Control: Insecticides, proper hygiene.
  Management and Control Measures: Quarantine: Quarantine new birds before introducing them to the flock. Sanitation: Regular cleaning and disinfection of poultry houses, equipment, and surroundings. Biosecurity: Implement strict biosecurity measures to prevent the introduction and spread of parasites. Deworming: Regular deworming programs using

effective anthelmintics. Insecticides: Application of insecticides to control external parasites. Vaccination: Utilize vaccines for specific internal parasites (e.g., coccidiosis).

VII. **Metabolic Disorders:** Metabolic disorders in poultry refer to conditions that affect the normal functioning of metabolic processes in birds. These disorders can have various causes, including nutritional imbalances, genetic factors, environmental stress, or management practices.

1. **Liver Dysfunction:** Liver dysfunction in poultry can result from various causes, including infectious diseases, toxins, nutritional imbalances, and metabolic disorders. The liver plays a crucial role in metabolism, digestion, and detoxification. When the liver is compromised, it can lead to a range of symptoms and negatively impact the overall health of the birds.

Causes

Infectious Diseases: Viral hepatitis (e.g., Infectious Bronchitis Virus, Adenovirus). Bacterial infections (e.g., Escherichia coli, Clostridium spp.). Protozoal infections (e.g., Histomonas meleagridis causing blackhead disease).

Toxins: Mycotoxins in feed (e.g., aflatoxins). Plant toxins (e.g., certain poisonous plants). Chemical toxins (e.g., exposure to pesticides or contaminants).

Nutritional Factors: Deficiency or imbalance of essential nutrients, especially vitamins and minerals. High-energy diets leading to fatty liver syndrome.

Metabolic Disorders: Fatty Liver Hemorrhagic Syndrome (FLHS) characterized by excessive fat accumulation in the liver.

Other metabolic imbalances affecting liver function.

Symptoms

Reduced Feed Intake: Birds may show decreased appetite.

Drop in Egg Production: In laying hens, a decline in egg production may occur.

Poor Growth and Weight Loss: Chicks or growing birds may exhibit poor growth rates.

Changes in Feces: Diarrhea or changes in fecal consistency.

Yellowing of Skin and Combs: Jaundice or yellowing of skin and combs may be visible in severe cases.

Neurological Signs: Neurological symptoms may occur, such as head shaking or tremors.

Ascites (Fluid Accumulation): Accumulation of fluid in the abdominal cavity (ascites) may occur.

Respiratory Distress: Birds may show signs of respiratory distress.

Diagnosis:

Clinical Signs: Observation of characteristic symptoms.

Blood Tests: Evaluation of liver enzymes and other blood parameters.

Post-mortem Examination: Necropsy may reveal liver lesions and abnormalities.

Prevention and Management:

Biosecurity Measures: Implement strict biosecurity to prevent the introduction of infectious agents.

Toxin Control: Monitor and control for mycotoxins and other toxins in feed.

Treatment

Treatment may involve addressing the underlying cause, supportive care, and administration of medications.

2. **Kidney Dysfunction:** Kidney dysfunction in poultry refers to conditions where the kidneys are compromised in their normal functioning. The kidneys play a crucial role in maintaining fluid balance, electrolyte balance, and excreting waste products from the body. Kidney dysfunction can be caused by various factors, including infectious agents, toxins, and metabolic disorders.

Causes

Infectious Diseases: Bacterial infections (e.g., Escherichia coli, Salmonella spp.). Viral infections (e.g., Infectious Bronchitis Virus, Newcastle Disease Virus).

Toxins: Mycotoxins in feed, such as ochratoxins. Exposure to environmental toxins or contaminants.

Metabolic Disorders: Gout, a condition characterized by the deposition of urate crystals in the kidneys. Nutritional imbalances affecting kidney function. Inadequate water supply or conditions leading to excessive water loss.

Symptoms

Increased Thirst, Birds may exhibit excessive drinking, Changes in Urination, Changes in urine volume, color, or consistency, Swollen Abdomen, Ascites or swelling in the abdominal region, Weight Loss, Reduced Activity, Lethargy or reduced activity levels, Changes in Feces, Changes in fecal color or consistency, Neurological symptoms may occur in severe cases.

Diagnosis

Clinical Signs: Observation of characteristic symptoms.

Blood Tests: Evaluation of kidney function parameters.

Post-mortem Examination: Necropsy may reveal kidney lesions and abnormalities.

Prevention and Management

Biosecurity Measures: Implement strict biosecurity to prevent the introduction of infectious agents.

Toxin Control: Monitor and control for mycotoxins and other toxins in feed and the environment.

Nutritional Management

Provide a balanced and properly formulated diet.

Proper Hydration: Ensure an adequate and clean water supply.

Treatment

Treatment may involve addressing the underlying cause, supportive care, and administration of medications.

3. **Gut Flora Impairment:** Gut flora impairment in poultry refers to disruptions or imbalances in the normal microbial communities (microbiota) residing in the gastrointestinal tract. The gut flora plays a crucial role in digestion, nutrient absorption, and overall gut health. Imbalances in the gut microbiota can result from various factors, including stress, infections, dietary changes, and the use of antibiotics.

   Causes

   Antibiotic Use: Broad-spectrum antibiotics can disrupt the balance of gut microbiota, leading to dysbiosis.

   Stress: Environmental stressors, such as high stocking density, transportation, or sudden changes in management practices, can impact gut health.

   Dietary Changes: Abrupt changes in diet or poor-quality feed can affect the composition of gut microbiota.

   Infections: Viral, bacterial, or parasitic infections can disturb the normal balance of gut microorganisms.

   Environmental Factors: Poor sanitation and suboptimal environmental conditions can contribute to the proliferation of harmful microorganisms.

   Immunosuppression: Conditions that suppress the immune system can increase susceptibility to gut flora imbalances.

   Symptoms

   Digestive Disturbances, Diarrhea or changes in fecal consistency, Reduced Feed Efficiency, Poor growth rates and reduced feed conversion, Higher mortality rates, especially in young birds. Weakened immune response, leading to increased susceptibility to other diseases. Reduced activity, lethargy, or signs of discomfort.

Diagnosis

Clinical Signs: Observation of characteristic symptoms.

Microbiota Analysis: Laboratory analysis of fecal samples to assess the composition of gut microbiota.

Prevention and Management

Use of probiotics (beneficial microorganisms) to promote a healthy gut microbiota. Inclusion of prebiotics in the diet to support the growth of beneficial microorganisms. Judicious use of antibiotics with consideration of their impact on gut microbiota.

Nutritional Management

Provide a balanced and high-quality diet to support gut health, Minimize stressors through proper management practices.

Treatment

Treatment may involve supportive care, dietary adjustments, and, in some cases, targeted antimicrobial therapy under veterinary guidance.

4. **Ascites:** Ascites in poultry is a condition characterized by the accumulation of fluid in the abdominal cavity. It is commonly observed in fast-growing meat-type chickens, especially broilers, and can lead to significant economic losses in poultry

production. Ascites is often associated with cardiovascular and respiratory issues, leading to increased pressure in the abdominal cavity.

Causes

Cardiovascular Issues: Rapid growth and high metabolic rates in modern broilers can strain the cardiovascular system, leading to heart failure. Constriction of blood vessels in the liver and other abdominal organs contributes to increased pressure in the abdominal cavity.

Respiratory Issues: Inadequate oxygen exchange in the lungs due to high metabolic demands can contribute to the development of ascites.

Genetic Factors: Some broiler strains are more prone to ascites due to genetic selection for rapid growth.

Symptoms

Accumulation of fluid leads to a distended abdomen (water belly).

Respiratory Distress: Labored breathing and increased respiratory rate.

Reduced Activity: Birds may exhibit lethargy and reduced mobility.

Increased Mortality: Ascites can lead to increased mortality rates, especially in affected birds.

Diagnosis

Clinical Signs: Observation of characteristic symptoms.

Necropsy: Post-mortem examination may reveal fluid accumulation in the abdominal cavity.

Prevention and Management

Genetic Selection: Select broiler strains with better cardiovascular and respiratory performance.

Ventilation and Environmental Management: Ensure proper ventilation and optimal environmental conditions.

Provide a well-balanced diet with consideration for energy levels and nutrient requirements.

Avoid overcrowding to reduce stress on the birds.

Treatment

Treatment options may include supportive care, nutritional adjustments, and, in severe cases, culling affected birds.

Understanding the types of poultry diseases and metabolic disorders is crucial for effective disease management and ensuring the health and well-being of poultry in commercial farming operations. Nutritional Deficiency in Poultry.

VIII. Nutritional Deficiencies

In poultry can have significant consequences, affecting growth, nutrient absorption, reproductive health, and immune function. Various vitamins and minerals are essential for maintaining poultry health. Here are some common nutritional deficiencies and their associated effects.

1. **Stunted Growth:** Stunted growth in poultry refers to a condition where birds exhibit slower-than-normal growth rates and fail to reach their expected size for their age. This can have various causes, including nutritional deficiencies, infectious diseases, environmental stress, and management issues. Identifying and addressing the underlying

factors contributing to stunted growth is crucial for optimizing flock performance.

Symptoms

Undersized Birds:Birds are smaller than expected for their age group.

Poor Feathering: Delayed or incomplete feather development.

Reduced Feed Efficiency: Poor feed conversion and lower weight gain.

Increased Mortality: Stunted birds may be more susceptible to diseases and have higher mortality rates.

Behavioral Changes: Lethargy, reduced activity, or abnormal behavior.

Diagnosis

Growth Monitoring: Regularly monitor flock growth performance.

Nutritional Analysis: Evaluate the nutrient content of the diet.

Health Assessment: Assess for signs of diseases or infections.

2. **Diminished Nutrients:** Diminished nutrients in poultry can refer to a situation where birds are not receiving an adequate or balanced supply of essential nutrients in their diet. Proper nutrition is critical for the growth, development, and overall health of poultry. Diminished nutrient levels can result from various factors, including poor-quality feed, imbalanced formulations, storage issues, or feed-related problems.

Causes

Poor-Quality Feed: Feed that is contaminated, spoiled, or of low quality may lack essential nutrients.

Imbalanced Formulations: Incorrect formulations or mixing errors in the feed manufacturing process can lead to imbalances in nutrient content.

Storage Issues: Improper storage conditions, such as exposure to moisture, heat, or pests, can degrade the quality of feed and reduce nutrient levels.

Feed Processing: Inadequate processing of feed ingredients can result in diminished nutrient availability.

Feed Additive Issues: Problems with the inclusion of vitamins, minerals, or other additives in the feed can impact nutrient levels.

Feed conversion ratios may be suboptimal. Nutrient

Symptoms

Birds may display specific symptoms of nutrient deficiencies, such as poor feathering, skeletal abnormalities, or developmental issues.

Lower Egg Production: In laying hens, diminished nutrient levels can lead to reduced egg production and poor egg quality.

Increased Mortality: Birds may be more susceptible to diseases and have higher mortality rates.

Behavioral Changes: Lethargy, reduced activity, or abnormal behavior.

Diagnosis:

Feed Analysis: Evaluate the nutrient content of the feed through laboratory analysis.

Nutritional Assessment: Examine birds for signs of nutrient deficiencies or imbalances.

Maintaining optimal nutrient levels in poultry diets is essential for achieving desired performance outcomes. Regular monitoring of feed quality, collaboration with a poultry nutritionist, and prompt action in case of suspected nutrient deficiencies are key elements in ensuring proper nutrition for poultry flocks.

IX. Impaired Reproductive Health:

Impaired reproductive health in poultry refers to conditions that negatively impact the reproductive organs and processes of birds, leading to reduced fertility, hatchability, or overall reproductive performance. Reproductive health is crucial for the sustainability of poultry flocks and the production of viable offspring. Several factors, including nutritional imbalances, infectious diseases, environmental stress, and genetic factors, can contribute to impaired reproductive health.

Symptoms

Impaired Reproductive Health

Reduced Egg Production: Decreased egg-laying rates or irregular laying patterns.

Poor Egg Quality: Eggs may have abnormalities in size, shape, or shell quality.

Low Fertility: Reduced fertility rates, leading to lower hatchability.

Embryonic Mortality: Increased rates of embryonic mortality during incubation.

Abnormal Reproductive Organs: Physical abnormalities or lesions in the reproductive organs.
Behavioral Changes: Changes in mating behavior, reduced courtship activities, or signs of distress.

Diagnosis

Reproductive Assessment: Evaluate reproductive organs and structures during post-mortem examinations.
Hormonal Analysis: Assess hormonal levels related to reproduction.
Egg Quality Testing: Analyze eggs for quality parameters.

Maintaining optimal reproductive health is essential for successful poultry breeding programs. Proactive management practices, regular veterinary checks, and attention to environmental and nutritional factors are key components in preventing and addressing issues related to impaired reproductive health in poultry flocks.

X. **Immune Suppression:** Immune suppression in poultry refers to a state where the normal functioning of the immune system is compromised, leading to reduced ability to mount an effective immune response against infections. A properly functioning immune system is crucial for protecting poultry against various pathogens, including bacteria, viruses, and parasites. Immune suppression can result from a variety of factors, and it poses a significant risk to the overall health and productivity of poultry flocks.

Symptoms

Increased Susceptibility to Infections: Birds become more prone to various infections.

Reduced Vaccine Efficacy: Vaccines may be less effective in poultry with a suppressed immune system.

Poor Growth and Performance: Immune-suppressed birds may exhibit slower growth rates and reduced overall performance.

Increased Mortality Rates:Higher mortality rates may occur due to an inability to combat infections.

Suboptimal Feed Conversion: Immune-suppressed birds may have poor feed efficiency.

Diagnosis

Clinical Signs: Observation of increased disease incidence, poor growth, or other signs of compromised health.

Laboratory Tests: Blood tests to assess immune parameters.

Efforts to prevent and manage immune suppression in poultry involve a combination of biosecurity measures, vaccination strategies, optimal nutrition, and environmental management. Early detection and intervention, along with collaboration with a poultry veterinarian, are critical for addressing immune suppression and maintaining the health and productivity of poultry flocks.

XI. **<u>Vitamin Deficiency</u>**

- **Vitamin A:** Symptoms include emaciation, reduced hatchability, embryonic mortality, keratinization of epithelial tissues, and ocular-nasal discharges. This deficiency is also known as Nutritional Roup.

- **Vitamin B1 (Thiamine):** Deficiency may cause polyneuritis, loss of appetite, nervous degeneration, lameness, and muscular paralysis.
- **Vitamin B2 (Riboflavin):** Symptoms include diarrhea, weakness, and a reduction in hatchability.
- **Vitamin B5 (Pantothenic Acid**): Deficiency may result in reduced egg production and embryonic hemorrhage.
- **Vitamin B6 (Pyridoxine):** Anemia, dermatitis, retarded growth, and chronic deficiency can lead to perosis.
- **Vitamin B7 (Biotin**): Deficiency can cause foot dermatitis, perosis, fatty liver, and kidney syndromes.
- **Vitamin E:** Essential for immunity and meat quality. Deficiency leads to diseases such as encephalomalacia (crazy chick disease), exudative diathesis, and muscular dystrophy.
- **Folic Acid (Folacin):** Anemia, tissue degeneration, and leukopenia are potential effects of deficiency.
- **Niacin (Nicotinic Acid):** Deficiency may lead to dermatitis, loss of appetite, stunted growth, and a lack of essential amino acids.
- **Vitamin B12 (Cobalamin):** Essential for enzymatic functions, deficiency can result

in loss of appetite, perosis, and nervous troubles.

- **Vitamin D3:** Also known as sunshine vitamin, it is crucial for calcium and phosphorus absorption. Deficiency leads to abnormal skeletal development, leg weakness, osteoporosis, and cracked eggshells.

XII. **Mineral Deficiencies:** Mineral deficiencies in poultry can occur when birds do not receive an adequate supply of essential minerals in their diet. Minerals play crucial roles in various physiological functions, including bone formation, enzyme activity, nerve function, and overall metabolic processes. Common minerals that are essential for poultry include calcium, phosphorus, magnesium, potassium, sodium, sulfur, trace minerals (such as iron, zinc, copper, manganese, selenium, and iodine), and others. Mineral deficiencies can lead to a range of health issues and negatively impact the performance and well-being of poultry.

Symptoms

Slow Growth Rates: Birds may exhibit poor growth performance.

Skeletal Abnormalities: Deformities in bones or joints. Poor Feathering, Dull or ragged feathers.

Reduced Egg Production: Decreased egg-laying rates, Soft or Thin Eggshells, Eggs may have poor shell quality.

Anemia: Pale comb, wattles, or mucous membranes.

Nervous Disorders: Tremors, weakness, or other neurological symptoms.

Muscular Dystrophy: Weakness in muscles.

- **Calcium and Phosphorus:** Essential for bone formation; deficiency can lead to conditions like rickets, cage layer fatigue, osteochondrosis, leg weakness, and reduced eggshell quality.
- **Magnesium:** Major role in eggshell and yolk formation; low egg production can result from its deficiency.
- **Iodine:** Controls thyroid hormone balance; deficiency leads to underactive thyroid activity and growth abnormalities.
- **Manganese:** Deficiency can result in perosis and chondrodystrophy, characterized by enlarged hock area, slipped tendons, and higher embryonic death rates.
- **Iron:** Essential to prevent anemia and reduce aflatoxin absorption.
- **Sodium, Chloride, and Potassium:** Important for maintaining osmoregulation and electrolyte balance.
- **Cobalt:** Deficiency leads to anemia and vitamin B12 deficiency.
- **Copper:** Symptoms include ataxia, spastic paralysis, leg weakness, and biochemical lesions in the aorta.
- **Zinc:** Responsible for various enzymatic actions; deficiency can cause poor growth, feathering issues, anorexia, and even mortality.
- **Selenium:** Plays an intrinsic role in the antioxidant system like vitamin E; deficiency leads to exudative diathesis.

Maintaining a well-balanced diet for poultry is crucial to prevent these nutritional deficiencies and ensure their overall health and productivity.

Addressing mineral deficiencies is essential for maintaining optimal health, growth, and reproductive performance in poultry. Neglecting mineral needs can lead to economic losses and welfare issues.

Mineral deficiencies should be addressed promptly through proper nutrition, supplementation, and regular monitoring. Collaborating with poultry nutritionists and veterinarians is crucial to developing effective strategies for preventing and managing mineral deficiencies in poultry flocks.

XIII. **Behavioral Disorders:** Behavioral disorders in poultry refer to abnormal or problematic behaviors exhibited by birds that deviate from typical or healthy patterns. These disorders can result from various factors, including genetic predisposition, environmental stressors, management practices, and health issues. Identifying and addressing behavioral disorders is crucial for ensuring the well-being of poultry flocks and optimizing their performance.

- Feather Pecking and Cannibalism: Birds peck at and pull out feathers of themselves or others. Cannibalism involves aggressive pecking leading to injuries.
  Causes: Crowded conditions, boredom, nutritional deficiencies, genetic predisposition, or environmental stress.
- Aggression and Dominance Behavior: Aggressive pecking or bullying, particularly in dominant birds towards subordinates.

Causes: Hierarchical disputes, overcrowding, resource competition, or inadequate socialization.

- Pacing or Circling: Continuous walking in circles or repetitive pacing.
  Causes: Stress, environmental monotony, or neurological issues.
- Nesting and Egg-Laying Disorders: Abnormal nesting behavior, egg eating, or laying eggs outside designated nests.
  Causes: Inadequate nest provision, environmental stress, or reproductive issues.
- Fear Responses and Shyness: Birds exhibit excessive fear responses, avoidance behaviors, or shyness.
  Causes: Poor handling practices, exposure to frightening stimuli, or genetic factors.
- Vocalization Disorders: Excessive or abnormal vocalizations, including constant loud calling or silence.
  Causes: Stress, environmental disturbances, or health issues.
- Agitated or Anxious Behavior: Restlessness, excessive preening, or other signs of agitation.
  Causes: Environmental stressors, changes in routine, or health concerns.
- Egg Eaters: Birds consume their own eggs.
  Causes: Nutritional deficiencies, inadequate nesting facilities, or learned behavior.
- Abnormal Dust Bathing: Birds may engage in excessive or abnormal dust bathing behaviors.
  Causes: Environmental factors, mite infestations, or stress.

- Isolation or Social Withdrawal: Birds may isolate themselves from the flock or exhibit antisocial behavior.
  Causes: Social stress, aggression, or health issues.

XIV. **Environmental Factors:**

- Heat Stress (Summer Stress): Poultry may experience heat stress during hot seasons, affecting their well-being. Proper management is crucial to mitigate the impact.
- Handling Stress: Stress induced by improper handling practices can adversely affect poultry. Ensuring gentle and careful handling is essential.
- Transportation Stress: The transportation process can subject poultry to stress. Adequate measures should be in place to minimize the negative effects.
- Traumatic Stress (Injury & Vaccinations): Traumatic stress, resulting from injuries or vaccinations, can impact poultry health. Careful procedures and post-care are essential to alleviate stress in such situations.

Addressing behavioral disorders is crucial for optimizing bird welfare, preventing injuries, and ensuring overall flock health and productivity.

Managing behavioral disorders in poultry requires a holistic approach, encompassing environmental, nutritional, and health considerations. Regular behavioral observation, preventive measures, and timely intervention contribute to the well-being and performance of poultry flocks.

HOMEOPATHIC APPROACHES TO POULTRY DISEASES

Homeopathy, recognized as an alternative system of medicine worldwide, extends its principles to the realm of poultry care. Poultry homeopathy is an integral part of veterinary homeopathy, emphasizing the similarities between principles applied in animals and humans, as articulated by Dr. Samuel Hahnemann in 1813.

Poultry birds share a substantial genetic resemblance to humans, with approximately 60 percent of chicken genes being analogous to human genes. Their anatomical systems, including Digestive, Respiratory, Skeletal, Muscular, Nervous, Circulatory, Endocrine, Excretory, Reproductive, and Immune Systems, closely mirror those of vertebrates. Notably, fowl lack a bladder; instead, their kidneys connect to ureters, opening into the cloaca, allowing the simultaneous excretion of urine and stool.

In the context of organic poultry farming, homeopathy emerges as a valuable alternative, offering a preventive regimen that enhances productivity within an economically viable range. The application of homeopathy ensures the exclusion of synthetic compounds from the poultry industry. This, in turn, contributes significantly to reducing Antibiotic Meat residues, combating antimicrobial drug resistance, and mitigating risks associated with hypersensitivity, carcinogenicity, mutagenicity, teratogenicity, and myelosuppression (inactive bone marrow). Such measures have a profound impact on the safety of the food supply chain and the overall healthcare management of the public.

Protocols for Poultry Health Care

Effectively managing poultry health requires a nuanced grasp of the subject along with skillful protocols. The shared health care protocols for poultry are rooted in personal experiences and keen observations, presenting a comprehensive strategy for addressing diseases, preventing issues, and providing supplementary care. It's important to recognize that individual circumstances may differ, and these protocols serve as a foundational guide.

A. Protocol for Treatment of the Disease:

Homeopathy, as a holistic system of medicine, focuses on addressing the root cause of diseases and stimulating the body's innate healing mechanisms. Below is a general outline of a homeopathic treatment protocol for poultry diseases:

1. Clinical Assessment: Conduct a thorough clinical assessment of the affected birds, considering symptoms such as behavior changes, respiratory distress, feed intake, and overall vitality.
2. Individualized Homeopathic Remedy Selection: Based on the observed symptoms, select individualized homeopathic remedies for the birds. Remedies are chosen considering not only the specific disease symptoms but also the unique constitution and characteristics of birds.
3. Potency and Dosage: Determine the appropriate potency and dosage of the selected homeopathic remedy. Potency selection is based on the severity and nature of symptoms, and dosage is adjusted according to the size and condition of the bird. Potencies: 30, 200, 3x, 12x, Dilution: 1 ml of medicine in 9 ml distilled water. Administration: 2 ml per bird. Duration: 3-5 consecutive days.

4. Observation and Adjustments: Regularly observe the birds for changes in symptoms and overall health. Adjust the homeopathic remedy or potency if necessary, based on the response to treatment.
5. Complementary Remedies: Consider complementary remedies or supportive treatments to address specific symptoms or complications associated with the disease.
6. Environmental and Nutritional Support: Implement environmental and nutritional improvements to support the overall health of the flock. This may include optimizing living conditions, providing proper nutrition, and ensuring access to clean water.
7. Record Keeping: Maintain detailed records of each bird's symptoms, treatment protocols, and responses. This information helps in assessing the effectiveness of homeopathic treatments over time.

B. Protocol for Disease Prevention:

Homeopathic preventive protocols for poultry diseases involve the use of homeopathic remedies to enhance the overall health and immunity of the flock, reducing the likelihood of disease outbreaks.

Explore homeopathic preventive measures, such as nosodes or constitutional remedies, to strengthen the birds' immune systems and reduce the risk of disease.

1. Constitutional Remedies: Administer constitutional homeopathic remedies based on the overall health and characteristics of the flock. These remedies aim to strengthen the birds' immune systems and promote resilience.
2. Nosodes: Introduce homeopathic nosodes, which are potentized substances derived from disease products. Nosodes are used to stimulate the immune system and provide specific protection against certain diseases.
3. Seasonal Adjustments: Adjust preventive measures seasonally, considering factors such as weather changes and environmental stressors. Homeopathic remedies can be tailored based on the specific challenges posed during different seasons.
4. Individualized Protocols: Develop individualized preventive protocols for each bird, considering factors like age, stress levels, and previous health history. This may involve periodic administration of homeopathic remedies to address underlying susceptibilities.
5. Prophylactic Use of Remedies: Consider the prophylactic use of certain homeopathic remedies

known for their general immune-boosting properties. Examples include Thuja, Silicea, and Calcarea carbonica.

6. Potency and Dosage: Identify the suitable potency and dosage for the chosen homeopathic remedy, with potency selection guided by the severity, freequency and nature of symptoms. Potencies: 200, 1M, Dilution: 1 ml of medicine in 9 ml distilled water, Administration: 2 ml per bird, Frequency: Weekly once.
7. Environmental Enhancements: Implement environmental enhancements to support the well-being of the flock. This includes maintaining clean and well-ventilated housing, optimizing nutrition, and providing access to fresh water.
8. Regular Observation & Record Keeping: Regularly observe the birds for any signs of stress or changes in behavior. Promptly address any emerging issues with appropriate homeopathic remedies. Maintain detailed records of preventive measures taken. This information aids in assessing the effectiveness of the preventive protocol.
9. Integration with Conventional Practices: Integrate homeopathic preventive measures with conventional biosecurity practices.

C. Protocols for Supplements:

A homeopathic supplementary protocol for poultry diseases involves using additional remedies and supportive measures to enhance the overall health and well-being of the flock, especially during or after disease challenges. This supplementary approach aims to provide additional support to the birds' immune systems and promote recovery. Here's a general outline for a homeopathic supplementary protocol.

1. Immune-Boosting Remedies: Administer homeopathic remedies known for their immune-boosting properties. Examples include Echinacea, Thuja, and Silicea. These remedies can support the birds' natural defense mechanisms.
2. Tonic Remedies: Introduce homeopathic tonic remedies to promote vitality and resilience. Ginseng, Avena sativa, and Alfalfa are examples of remedies that may be considered for overall well-being.
3. Detoxification Support: Include homeopathic remedies with detoxifying properties to help the birds eliminate any lingering toxins. Nux vomica and Sulphur are potential options to consider.
4. Stress Management: Administer remedies that address stress-related symptoms. These may include Argentum nitricum, Gelsemium, or other remedies tailored to the specific stressors affecting the flock.
   Recovery Support: Provide homeopathic remedies that support the recovery process after a disease outbreak. Arnica, China, and Phosphorus are examples that may assist in the restoration of vitality.

5. Individualized Protocols: Develop individualized supplementary protocols for each bird, taking into account their unique constitution and response to previous treatments.
6. Nutritional Enhancements: Consider homeopathic remedies that address nutritional deficiencies or imbalances. These remedies may complement dietary adjustments to optimize nutrition.
7. Environmental Considerations: Evaluate the homeopathic remedies that can positively influence the birds' response to environmental challenges. Remedies such as Pulsatilla or Natrum muriaticum might be considered based on observed behaviors.

These homeopathic protocols are designed for the effective treatment, prevention, and supplementation of poultry care. The specified potencies and dilutions, along with recommended administration frequencies, aim to address various health aspects in poultry birds, promoting their well-being and minimizing the risk of diseases. It is advisable to adhere to the outlined guidelines for optimal results.

ENHANCING POULTRY HEALTH THROUGH HOMEOPATHIC SOLUTIONS

Revolutionize your poultry farming practices with the transformative power of homeopathic solutions. Discover a holistic approach to enhancing poultry health, focusing on natural remedies and preventive measures. Elevate your poultry management strategies with the gentle yet effective touch of homeopathy, promoting overall well-being and reducing the reliance on synthetic compounds. Embrace a new era in poultry health management through homeopathic solutions.

1. Prophylaxis Care

In the realm of homeopathic solutions, prophylaxis care is a methodical and preventative approach designed to uphold the health and well-being of poultry. This approach strategically employs specific remedies and treatments with the aim of not only minimizing the risk of diseases but also bolstering overall immunity in poultry.

- Nosodes: Tailored remedies derived from disease-causing agents, recommended for specific illnesses. Utilized in poultry management to proactively reduce disease prevalence.
- Thuja Occidentalis: A versatile remedy with anti-sycotic and anti-viral properties. Beneficial for respiratory tract infections, bronchitis, and immune modulation.

- Maladrinum: Mitigates adverse effects of vaccinations and addresses issues like fowl pox and nodular skin lesions.
- Streptococcinum: Effectively combats acute septicemia, cellulitis, and various infections.
- Aviaire: Excellent for managing influenza, loss of strength, and appetite.
- Bacillus Subtile: Supports gut and intestinal health, contributing to autoimmune correction.
- Sulphur: An anti-psoric remedy valuable when the initially selected remedy proves ineffective.
- Nux Vomica: A significant polycrest remedy known for managing drug resistance and chronic health derangements.
- Calcarea Carb: A constitutional remedy with profound effects, enhancing normal body functions.

2. Adequate Nutrition

Enhance your poultry nutrition strategy by incorporating a range of vital homeopathic remedies. The homeopathic method for ensuring optimal nutrition in poultry revolves around the targeted use of specific remedies. This approach is designed to tackle deficiencies, stimulate optimal growth, and elevate the overall well-being of the flock.

- Calcarea Phos: Tackles calcium or phosphorus deficiency, rickets, and aids in osteophyte restoration.
- Selenium: Beneficial for exudative diathesis, bone health, and addressing sexual atony.
- Silicea: Enhances assimilation, supports bone health, and counteracts the adverse effects of vaccination.

- Alfa Alfa: Acts as a weight gainer and appetizer.
- Cypripedium Pubescens: Functions as a nerve tonic.
- Iodium: Addresses impaired metabolism, poor growth, and enhances phagocytic actions.
- Mangnum Phosphoricum: Stabilizes normal CNS functions and aids in phosphorus utilization.
- Phosphorous: Enhances organic compound metabolism.
- Xanthoxylum Fraxineum: Addresses poor assimilation and indigestion.
- Strontium Iodatum: Useful for addressing low iodine levels.
- Galega Officinalis: Addresses impaired nutrition and acts as an appetite enhancer.
- Lipoicum Acidum: Enhances growth and provides powerful antioxidant properties.
- Acidum Molybdenum: Boosts hormonal activities.
- Aurum Ars: Increases appetite.

3. Anti-Stress

Incorporate targeted homeopathic remedies to alleviate stress-related symptoms and enhance the overall well-being of poultry in the anti-stress homeopathic solution for poultry.

- Arsenic Album: Effective against higher viral loads and anxiety.
- Passiflora: Useful for acute manias, anxiety, and poor nutrition.
- Beta Vulgaris: Possesses antioxidant, nephro-protective, and anti-inflammatory properties.
- Aconite: Anxiolytic remedy effective against anxiety, heat stress, and sudden shock.

- Carbo Vegs: Useful for respiratory acidosis, imperfect oxidation, and improving vitality.
- Acid Phos: Acts on the nervous system, promoting mental and physical well-being.
- Acidum Ascorbicum: A potent antioxidant.
- Ignatia: Effective for post-traumatic stress and stress-induced complaints.
- Lobelia Inflata: Acts on pneumo-gastric and vasomotor functions.
- Natrum Sulph: An electrolyte re-loader.
- Cydonia Vulgaris: An energy tonic.
- Five Phos Bio Chemic: Maintains mineral and electrolyte balance.
- Achillea Millifolium: Useful for high temperatures, overexertion, and severe hemorrhages.

4. Mycotoxins

The homeopathic solution for Mycotoxins in poultry involves using specific remedies to counteract the harmful effects of mycotoxin exposure and promote overall health in birds.

- Carbo Vegetabilis: Aids in removing toxins from the body and prevents toxemia.
- Lycopodium: Enhances kidney and liver functions, minimizing hepatic lesions.
- Carthamus Tinctorius: Activates enzymatic actions and supports the immune response.
- Terminalia Chebula: Anti-neurotoxic and inhibits the growth of intestinal pathogenic bacteria.
- Kalmegh: A liver remedy and blood purifier.

- Berberis Vulgaris: Addresses kidney impairment, reduces liver enzyme activity, and controls metabolic disorders.
- Silibum Marianum: Prevents mycotoxins and promotes liver health.
- Embolia Officinalis: A liver protector and immune modulator.
- Lufffa Amara: A liver tonic.
- Veratrum Album: Addresses toxemia.
- Nux Vomica: A significant polycrest remedy effective against drug resistance and chronic health derangements.
- Kali Hypo Phosphoricum: Addresses impaired kidneys and acts as an anti-stress agent, reducing plasma phosphate.
- Chimphilia: A lymphatic stimulant that enhances immunity.
- Serum Musa Acuminata: Effective against chronic kidney disorders and deficiencies in calcium and magnesium.
- Yucca: An antioxidant that prevents oxidative stress and provides liver support.
- Ceanothus Americanus: Hepato-protective and regenerative.

5. Infectious Diseases

Homeopathic solutions for infectious diseases in poultry have a dual focus: alleviating symptoms, boosting the immune system, and supporting overall health to combat specific pathogens. It is crucial to note that preventing, managing, and controlling infectious diseases necessitate guidance from healthcare professionals.

6. Metabolic and Nutritional Disorders

Homeopathic solutions for metabolic and nutritional disorders in poultry are dedicated to rectifying imbalances, deficiencies, and fostering overall health. This approach involves the implementation of strategies such as health and immunity enhancement, organ improvement therapies, supplementation, gut health promoters, appetizers, and blood purifiers.

7. Behavioral and Environmental Disorders

Homeopathic solutions for behavioral and environmental disorders in poultry are designed to target diverse psychological and stress-related challenges faced by birds in their surroundings. The management involves the application of constitutional medicine and anti-stress therapies tailored to address issues like cannibalism and depression, with the selection of remedies based on symptom similarities.

HOMEOPATHIC APPROACH TO MAJOR POULTRY DISEASES

Viral Infections

Effectively managing viral infections in breeder and broiler birds in the poultry industry involves a comprehensive approach focusing on prevention, early detection, and appropriate treatment strategies. Here are key aspects to consider:

Preventive Measures: Vaccination Protocols: Implement a robust vaccination schedule tailored to the specific viral threats prevalent in the region. This includes vaccinations against diseases such as Newcastle Disease, Infectious Bronchitis, Avian Influenza, and others.

Biosecurity Practices: Establish stringent biosecurity measures to prevent the introduction and spread of viruses. This includes restricted access, hygiene protocols, and proper disposal of litter and carcasses.

Quarantine Procedures: Introduce a thorough quarantine system for new birds entering the facility to identify and isolate any potential carriers of viral infections before they can spread to the existing flock.

Early Detection: Regular Monitoring: Implement routine monitoring programs, including clinical observation and laboratory testing, to detect any signs of viral infections early on.

Diagnostic Tools: Utilize advanced diagnostic tools such as PCR tests and serological assays for accurate and timely identification of viral pathogens.

Treatment and Management: Antiviral Medications: In cases where viral infections are diagnosed, consider the use of antiviral medications if available and deemed effective against the specific virus.

Supportive Care: Provide supportive care to affected birds, including proper nutrition, hydration, and maintaining optimal environmental conditions to help them cope with the infection.

Culling Strategy: Depending on the severity and type of viral infection, develop a culling strategy to remove affected birds and prevent further spread within the flock.

1. Newcastle Disease/ND (Renikhet Disease/RD)

Newcastle disease is a highly contagious and often fatal viral infection in the poultry industry, with mortality rates ranging from 50-100%. While there is no specific treatment, antibiotics are used to control secondary infections. Prevention involves vaccination, stringent quarantine measures, and effective biosecurity and sanitary practices.

Indications: Caused by paramyxovirus, avian orthoavulavirus 1, a negative-sense, single-stranded RNA virus. Initial symptoms include mild respiratory issues like gasping, sneezing, and coughing. Progresses to bronchitis and neurological manifestations such as depression, weakness, muscular spasm, tremors, paralysis, twisted head & neck (torticollis), acute death, facial edema, diarrhea, loss of appetite, drop in egg production, and drooped wings with ruffled feathers. Four common symptomatic manifestations based on pathogenicity are lentogenic ND, mesogenic ND, neurotropic velogenic ND, and viscerotropic velogenic ND.

Homeopathic Medicinal Management

- Belladonna: Addresses inflammations, prevents damage to the central nervous system, and aids in air sickness.
- Cicuta Virosa: Anti-viral properties, particularly effective for torticollis and spine deformities.
- Arsenicum Album: Alleviates difficulty breathing, provides anti-viral support to respiratory cells, addresses greenish discharges, and enhances vitality.
- Kali Phos: Nerve remSedy useful for prostration, neurasthenia, depression, and promotes cell growth and repair.
- Hypericum: Anti-viral support for mild paralysis and respiratory symptoms associated with neurological symptoms.
- Aconite: Addresses mental and physical restlessness, fever, acute and sudden illness, and provides anti-viral support.
- Carbo Veg: Improves vitality, addresses imperfect oxidation, and counters toxemia.
- Veratrum Album: Addresses greenish watery stool with prostration.
- Gelsemium: Effective for muscular weakness, trembling, paralysis, CNS stimulation, respiratory illness, and anti-viral support during heat stress.
- Mag Phos: Addresses twisting neck (torticollis), provides pain relief, anti-spasmodic properties, and aids emaciated animals with cramps and spasms.

- Capsicum Annum: Useful for weakness, myalgia, nerve damage, induces immunity reactions, and serves as an alternative for antibiotic growth promoters (AGP).
- Nigella Sativa: Enhances immunity during viral challenges, reduces viral load, and pro-inflammatory mediators. Promotes IgG1 and IgG2a levels in serum.

2. Infectious Bursal Disease (Gumboro)

Infectious Bursal Disease (IBD), commonly known as Gumboro, is an acute viral infection affecting young chickens and is caused by the IBD virus, an RNA virus. The poultry birds are predominantly affected by Sero type-1 of the virus, leading to immune suppression and increased mortality generally occurring between 3 to 6 weeks of age. The bursa fabricus (Bursa cloacalis), a specialized organ located in the posterior part of the cloaca, is primarily responsible for immunity, particularly for B-cell development.

Indications: IBD virus hampers the development of the birds' immune system, resulting in a mortality rate of 50-60%. IBD infection manifests as inflammation followed by atrophy of the bursa. Symptoms include immune suppression, prostration, debilitation, dehydrated birds, unsteady gait, watery diarrhea with a swollen vent, vent pecking, inappetence (anorexia), and nephrosis.

Homeopathic Medicinal Management

- Calendula: Boosts immunity through lymphatic drainage stimulation, acts as a hepatic protector, and exhibits anti-microbial and anti-viral properties.
- Mentha piperita: Possesses anti-viral properties and supports T-cell and cytokine production.
- Aconitum napellus: Addresses anxiety and restlessness, particularly effective for acute illnesses, acts as an anti-viral agent, and helps with inflammations. Suitable for ailments triggered by winter and cold.
- Gelsemium: Acts in the brain to alleviate pain, especially effective for neuralgic affections, and can be beneficial for conditions like measles and pellagra.
- Echinacea angustifolia: Effective in acute auto infections, serves as a corrector of blood poisonings, and is particularly useful for virulent infections and lymphatic inflammations.
- Medicago Sativa: Possesses biological activities and promotes appetite, especially beneficial for individuals with rheumatic diathesis.
- Acidum Phosphoricum: Promotes mental and physical well-being, aiding in preventing fatigue and stress.
- X-RAY: Enhances cellular metabolism.
- Ferrum phos: Acts as an antipyretic, especially effective for acute infections.
- Calcarea phos: Serves as a calcium source, promoting bone health, providing solidity to bones, and acting as a nutritive remedy for periosteum and

bones. Helpful in bone diseases and blood deficiencies.

- Melissa Officinalis: Exhibits anti-inflammatory and anti-spasmodic properties.
- Tinospora cordifolia: Acts as an immune modulator.

INDICATIONS	COMPLICATIONS	PROTOCOL
IBD virus (RNA virus) Sero type 1 viruses Infectious Bursitis, Avian nephrosis	Narcotizing the cells, Acute death, Severe mortality. Hepatic degeneration,	Anti-Viral, Lymphatic stimulant, Hepatic protector.
Neuronal Degeneration CNS Depression	Degenerate the nerve cells Impaired immune system, Acute Death.	Neuronal protector, Anxiolytic, Anti-inflammatory
Immune suppression Vaccination failure	Prevent and destruct the development of lymphoid follicle in Bursa.	Immune Modulator
Watery diarrhea with swollen vent, Vent pecking.	Low feed intake, Weight loss, Weakness, Dehydration, Stress, Weight loss, Dyspepsia.	Weight Gainer, Metabolizer, Appetizer

3. Inclusion Body Hepatitis (IBH)

Also known as Hepatitis Hypopericardium Syndrome, IBH is caused by fowl adenovirus in young avian species, with sudden mortality typically observed in the 6th week of age. There is no specific treatment for IBH infections, and for prevention, both live and inactive vaccines are available.

Indications: IBH virus-infected birds exhibit lethargy, anorexia, mucoid droppings due to excess bile, inflamed and enlarged liver with hemorrhagic spots, and yellowish discoloration of the liver. Hepatic cell necrosis is a characteristic feature. IBH is transmitted both horizontally and vertically, with the prevention of vertical transmission being an effective prophylactic measure.

Both live and inactive vaccines are available to reduce infection rates, and some antibiotics may help prevent secondary infections.

Homeopathic Medicinal Management:

- Nux vomica: Addressing hepatitis symptoms based on similarity.
- Podophyllum: Effective for indigestion and gastroenteritis, acting on the liver and intestines.
- Lycopodium: Useful for hepatitis, anti-stress, ascites, and simultaneous action on the liver and kidneys.
- Oleum jecoris aselli: A hepatic and pancreatic remedy with benefits for scrofulous affections.
- Chelidonium: Promotes enzymatic actions, exhibits anti-tumor and genotoxic activity, and is a prominent liver remedy.
- Mirabilis Jalappa: Acts as a hepatic protector.

- Kalmegh: Exhibits antiviral properties, enhances liver functions, and has anti-oxidative and anti-inflammatory effects.
- Berberis aristata: Protective, anti-hepatomegaly, anti-hepatotoxic, and effective for jaundice and fever.
- Silybium marianus: A hepatic protector that promotes hepatic cell regeneration.
- Embolia officinalis: Immunomodulatory, hepatoprotective, anti-fibrotic, and exhibits antiviral properties.
- Lycopodium clavatum: A poly-chrest remedy effective for hepatotoxicity, impaired liver functions, and blood circulations.
- Calcarea Sulph: Acts on the liver and bile, serving as a pH regulator and blood purifier.
- Achillea millefolium: Useful for hemorrhages and as a hepatic stimulator.
- Swertia Chirata: Addresses liver diseases, bile disorders, and acts as a blood purifier.
- IBH Nosode

4. Chicken Anemia Virus (CAV)

It is a single stranded DNA virus. Disease characterized Aplastic anemia, Bone marrow atrophy and Lymphoid atrophy associated immune suppression especially affected in young birds.

Indications: Cyanosis, Weakness, Paleness in comb, wattle, legs and eyelids. This disease also known as blue wing disease and Anemia dermatitis syndrome.

Homeopathic Medicinal Management

- Ferrum metalicum - Anemic, Cyanosis, Irregular blood distribution, Impaired blood circulations.
- Ferrum phos - Increase Hb, pale and anemia.
- Lecithin - RBC modulation.
- Medicago Sativa - As a tonic, Supplementary aid.
- Echinacea - Immune stimulant, Blood poisoning.
- Ferrum citricum - Deficiency anemia, iron storage disorders.
- Withenia somnifera - Prevent virus multiplication.
- Hyocyamus niger - Viral Toxemia.
- Calcarea arsenicosum - Low Hemoglobin and RBC count.
- Prunus virginiana – Blood Tonic.

5. Avian influenza

Highly fatal infectious disease caused by family Orthomyxovirus viridae, it will transmit to human from infected birds, yearly 3-5 million are cases are reporting, Infections leads high fever, cough, loss of appetite, head ache and fatigues. Mainly Avian influenza virus are classified into the two categories based on their grade of pathogenicity.

1. **Low Pathogenic Avian Influenza (LPAI)** – Type A Orthomyxoviridae. Mild signs relating to the respiratory, alimentary.

2. **Highly Pathogenic Avian Influenza (HPAI)** – H5N1 virus. Depressed, Egg production falls and soft-shelled eggs, Watery diarrhea, respiratory signs, swelling of the face.

Indications: - Avian Influenza infected birds manifested Edema in Head (comb and wattles), Cyanosis of wattle, comb, leg etc., diarrhea, nasal discharge, coughing and sneezing, soft shelled egg, pinpoint hemorrhage on feet and shank, Mild sinusitis.

Homeopathic Medicinal Management

- Influenzinum - Influenzas Bronchitis, Cold, Catarrh and influenza, Prophylaxis case, Sneezing, Sinusitis.
- Allium cepa - Useful in initial stage of flu (cough and sneezing), Heat in different part of body (comb & Wattles), profuse watery nasal discharge, Hay fever, Sneezing, Neuralgic pains.
- Arsenicum album- Remedy for respiratory system and anti-viral, Seasonal complaints.
- Kali iod - Watery, acrid coryza, glandular swellings, worse in cold, Associated Bacterial and fungi infections present.
- Belladonna - Anti-inflammatory, Sudden onset of fever and cough and cold.
- Drosera - Laryngeal phthisis with irritation and profuse expectoration, Helps clear out the respiratory tract.
- Gelsemium - Anti viral, helps to control neurological abnormalities.
- Aconite - Acute manifestation, Fever, Stress.
- Millifolium - High temperature with mild influenza symptoms.
- Sambacus nigra – Helps to prevent cold and flu symptoms, Boost your immune system, Anti stress.

6. Egg Dropping Syndrome (EDS)

EDS caused by Atadeno virus, Clinical signs in layer birds are soft shelled egg in healthy birds, Egg drops may be 5-50%, loss of egg pigments. Ovian follicles broken, infections also present. characterized by the production of soft-shelled and shell-less eggs.

Indications: Drop in Egg Production, Soft-Shelled or Shell-Less Eggs, Decreased Shell Quality, Changes in Egg Appearance, Respiratory Signs, Depression and Lethargy, Drop in Feed Consumption, Increased Mortality.

Homeopathic Medicinal Management

- Calcarea carb - Calcium intake & absorption stability.
- Calcarea phos - As a calcium source, Improve egg quality.
- Silicea - Improve nutritional absorption.
- Pulsatilla nigricans - Synchronize ovarian functions.
- Medicago Sativa - Rich with amino acids, Vitamins, tocopherol and Estrogen.
- Folliculinum – Drainage remedy to stimulate ovulation.
- Natrum carb – Helps for the retention of sperm.
- Medorrhinum – Miasmatic remedy.
- Thuja – Ailments from Suppressive drug therapy.
- Withenia Somnifera – Helps to re-correct hormonal abnormalities.

BACTERIAL INFECTIONS

Bacterial infections in poultry manifest in a multitude of ways, affecting different systems and organs within birds. The range of severity varies, from mild to severe, and has significant implications for the overall health and productivity of the flock. Tackling bacterial infections in poultry is a complex task, posing considerable challenges to both farmers and the poultry industry at large. Successfully managing these challenges requires a comprehensive and integrated approach. This includes implementing stringent biosecurity measures to prevent disease spread, devising strategic vaccination plans to enhance flock immunity, adhering to sound management practices, and ensuring prompt veterinary interventions when needed. Adopting such a holistic strategy is pivotal for maintaining the health and well-being of poultry populations and sustaining the industry's productivity.

Antibiotic resistance in poultry has emerged as a significant concern, posing threats to both animal health and human well-being. The indiscriminate use of antibiotics in conventional farming practices has contributed to the development of resistant strains of bacteria. As a result, exploring alternative, sustainable solutions, such as homeopathy, has gained prominence.

Complications of Antibiotic Use:

- Resistant Strains: Prolonged use of antibiotics leads to the evolution of resistant bacterial strains, reducing the effectiveness of conventional treatments.

- Residue Buildup: Antibiotic residues in poultry products can find their way into the human food chain, potentially causing health complications.

Opportunities with Homeopathic Medicine:

- Organic and Sustainable: Homeopathic solutions align with organic poultry farming practices, providing a sustainable and ethical approach to disease management.
- Reduced Antibiotic Dependency: Homeopathy aims to minimize reliance on antibiotics, offering an alternative that doesn't contribute to the development of resistant strains.
- Holistic Health: Homeopathic remedies focus on holistic well-being, addressing underlying health imbalances and boosting the immune system.

Some of the Challenges as follows:

- Disease Spread and Transmission: Bacterial infections can spread rapidly within a flock, leading to increased morbidity and mortality rates.
- Antibiotic Resistance: Development of antibiotic-resistant strains of bacteria poses a significant challenge in poultry farming. Overuse or misuse of antibiotics can contribute to the emergence of resistant strains.
- Impact on Production Efficiency: Bacterial infections can lead to reduced feed efficiency, slower growth rates, and decreased egg production, impacting overall production efficiency.
- Economic Losses: Outbreaks of bacterial infections can result in economic losses due to increased

mortality rates, treatment costs, and decreased productivity.

- Vaccine Development and Efficacy: Developing effective vaccines against bacterial pathogens can be challenging, and vaccine efficacy may vary.
- Diagnostic Challenges: Accurate and timely diagnosis of bacterial infections is crucial for effective disease management. However, diagnostics may be challenging, especially in the early stages of infection.
- Public Health Concerns: Some bacterial pathogens in poultry can pose risks to human health, especially through the food chain.
- Zoonotic infections and the presence of antibiotic-resistant bacteria are public health concerns.

Challenges and Considerations:

- Education and Awareness: Overcoming skepticism and enhancing awareness about homeopathy's efficacy is crucial.
- Integration with Conventional Practices: Integrating homeopathy into existing poultry management practices requires careful consideration and collaboration with veterinary professionals.
- Homeopathy presents an opportunity to address antibiotic resistance in poultry by offering an alternative that prioritizes organic, sustainable practices and emphasizes holistic health. As the poultry industry explores solutions to mitigate the impact of antibiotics, homeopathy stands out as a promising avenue for promoting the health and welfare of poultry flocks.

1. Collibacilosis (E-coli infections)

Avian pathogenic Escherichia coli (APEC) is the primary cause of colibacillosis in poultry. Higher mortality rates (30–35%), In the case of E-coli management in poultry multi drug resistance is the biggest challenge facing the industry. Proper water Sanitation and Antibiotic therapy are the treatment protocols for the Escherichia Coli infection. Frequency use of antibiotic usage will lead to antibiotic resistance.

Indications: E-coli infection will lead to septicemia, sub-acute air Scaulits and cellulitis as well as less productivity and different syndromes like yolk sac infection, omphalitis, respiratory tract infection, swollen head syndrome.

Medicinal Management

- Bacilinum - Indicated lung affections, Bronchorrhoea, Respiratory pyorrhea, Pneumonia.
- Drosera - Laryngeal phthisis, Vomiting food, Profuse expectoration.
- Ipecacuanha - Action over Pneumogastric nerve, nausea vomiting, Indicated after indigestible food, Moist weather.
- Influenzinum - Respiratory viral Infection.
- Pyrogenium - Septic infections.
- Thuja - Anti bacterial, Bird flu) It Will helps to increase oxidative metabolism of birds.
- E-Coli Nosode - E-Coli infections, Helps for prevention. Escherichia Coli – E-coli infection, Nosode.
- Aspidospermia - Stimulate pneumatic Centre, Increase oxygen to blood.
- Oscillococcinum – Birds flu.

- Strepto coccinum – Bacterial Infections.
- Ferrum phosphoricum - Acute infections, emaciation, Prostration, Bronchitis.
- Nux vomica – Polychrest remedy, Bad effects of antibiotic and vaccines.
- Avena Sativa – Bacteremia (Staph and E-coli Infections).
- Rauwolfia serpentina – Anti bacterial property against E-Coli infections.

2. Necrotic Enteritis

The overgrowth of Clostridium perfringens in the small intestine of broiler chickens, particularly during the 2nd to 6th weeks of age, is associated with a condition known as necrotic enteritis. Necrotic enteritis is a bacterial disease that can have significant economic impacts on the poultry industry due to increased mortality, reduced growth rates, and the costs associated with prevention and treatment. Here's an explanation of the key aspects of Clostridium perfringens overgrowth in broiler chickens:

Indications: Pathogens collapse the intestinal walls, it will lead to hemorrhage and reductions in the digestions and absorption of nutrients, Necrotic intestine, Increase mortality, Diarrhea and wet litter, Low feed conversion ratio, Intestinal catarrh.

Medicinal Management

- Nux vomica - Anti diarrheal. Anti-inflammatory, Promote digestion. Intestinal catarrh.
- Condurango - Recorrect the digestive functions, stimulates gastric secreations and improve Intestinal Health.

- Arsenicum album – Feed Toxins, Dyspepsia.
- Cuprum arsenicosum - Enteroptosis, Diarrhea and Dysentery.
- China - Disordered appetite, intestinal hemorrhage, Peritonitis.
- Mercurius corro - Anti ulcerative, amoebic dysentery, Anti-microbial.
- Alfalfa - Appetizer and digestion, malnutrition.
- Ornithogalum - Enteritis, Gastric disturbances, Chronic gastritis Enhance gastric health.
- Veratrum album - Anti diarrheal, Hyperemia, cholera asiatica. Gastric catarrh, Extreme weakness.
- Solanum nigrum - Chronic Intestinal toxicity.
- Holarrhena pubesscens - Anti Dysenteric.

3. Infectious Coryza

An acute respiratory disease caused by the avian bacterium Avibacterium paragallinarum is characterized by symptoms such as sneezing, sinusitis in the infraorbital region, ocular and nasal discharges, facial swelling, and a subsequent reduction in productivity.

Indications: Respiratory Signs: Sneezing, Coughing, Nasal discharge, swelling of the face and infraorbital sinuses, giving birds a characteristic "swollen head" appearance, Watery eyes, Swollen conjunctiva, Infected layers may experience a drop-in egg production. The presence of a foul odor is sometimes associated with the disease.

Medicinal Management

- Arsenicum album - Anti viral infections like flu, Respiratory troubles.
- Alliumcepa - Coryza, First stage of infections, watery nasal discharges.
- Influenzinum - Cold, Catarrh, Coryza, Preventive remedy.
- Sabadilla - Action over mucous membrane, cold, hay fever, diarrhea.
- Rumex - Cough, Inflammations, Lymphatic swellings.
- Pulsatilla - Yellow greenish discharges, Reduced water intake, droppings.
- Mercurius vivus - Worse from damp cold rainy weather, prostrations and trembling, greenish, bloody droppings.
- Hepar sulphur - Profuse secretions, vitamin B3 Deficiency, diarrhea.
- Euphrasia officinalis - Conjunctivitis, profuse lachrymation, bland coryza.
- Aconitum napellus - Acute remedy, fever, hot weather, influenza, hyperemia.

4. Fowl Cholera

The common acute disease caused by the gram-negative rod bacteria Pasteurella multocida is typically associated with a range of clinical symptoms affecting poultry. The infection manifests with various signs, indicating its impact on multiple organ systems. Here is an explanation of the clinical manifestations associated with Pasteurella multocida infection.

Indications: Affected birds exhibit a loss of appetite, leading to reduced or complete cessation of food intake. The presence of fever is indicated by an elevated body temperature, a common response to infection. Infected birds may experience profuse and watery diarrhea, contributing to dehydration, bluish discoloration of the skin and mucous membranes, may occur due to respiratory distress and compromised oxygenation. Birds may excrete droppings with a yellowish tint, reflecting changes in liver function or bile pigment metabolism. Visible swelling in the wattles, comb, joints, and feet is indicative of inflammation and edema associated with the infection.

Birds may exhibit nasal discharges, indicating respiratory involvement and inflammation of the nasal passages.Swellings beneath the mandible (sub-mandibular) may occur, suggesting lymph node involvement and localized inflammation.

Medicinal Management

- Sulphur - Anti-psoric, prostration, offensive discharges.
- Anti-tart - Respiratory illness, rattling mucous, Drowsiness, Bloody mucus stool.
- Camphora - Weak, Prostration, Rice Watery Diarrhea, Dehydration.
- Ferrum phos - Acute Infections and Fever.
- Carbo vegeteblis - Severe prostration, Collapsive stage, Panting.
- Veratrum album - Extreme Prostration, Hyperaemia, Greenish Diarrhea.

5. Avian Tuberculosis

Infections caused by Mycobacterium avium in poultry can result in a range of clinical signs and symptoms, impacting both the overall health and productivity of the affected birds. Here is an explanation of the manifestations associated with Mycobacterium avium infections.

Indications: Birds infected with Mycobacterium avium may experience significant weight loss due to the impact of the infection on the digestive and metabolic processes. Diarrhea is a common clinical sign, contributing to dehydration and further weight loss. Lameness may occur as a result of joint and skeletal involvement, with the bacteria affecting the musculoskeletal system. Infected birds often exhibit signs of depression, characterized by lethargy, reduced activity, and a general lack of interest in their surroundings. Mycobacterium avium infections can lead to pulmonary lesions, affecting the respiratory system. Birds may exhibit respiratory distress and other respiratory symptoms.

Medicinal Management

- Aviaire - Action over the lung, Bronchitis, Cold, Catarrh, helps to improve appetite.
- Phosphorous - Mucous membrane degeneration, inflamed serous membranes, Hemorrhage, weight loss, loss appetite, neuritis, inflamed respiratory tract.
- Stannum metalicum - Action over the respiratory organs, chronic lung complaints, tubercular diathesis.
- Acalypha indica - Bloody expectoration, Progressive weight loss.

- Tuberculinum - Nosode remedy, Emaciation.
- Arsenicum album - Poly-chrest remedy, Remedy for respiratory system and anti-viral, Seasonal complaints.
- Veratrum album - Extreme Prostration, Hyperemia, Greenish Diarrhea.
- Calcarea carbonicum – Developing stage.
- Calcarea Sulphuric – Yellowish mucoid discharges, Cutaneous tuberculosis, skin lesions with nodular appearance.
- Copaiva Officinalis – Early stage, well-marked nettle rashes.
- Stannum metalicum – Purulent discharges, Weakness.
- Dictamus albus – Helps to control respiratory troubles like flu and cold, Expectorant, Anti septic property.
- Ipecacuanha – Action over the pneumogastric nerve.
- Justicia adathoda – Catarrhal conditions of respiratory tract, Control excessive cough and dyspnoea.
- Lobelia inflata – Vasomotor stimulant, Bronchitis.
- Glycyrrhiza glabra – Expectorant, Cough, Antiulcer.

6. Pullorum Disease

Bacillary White Diarrhea, also known as Pullorum Disease, is a bacterial infection in poultry caused by Salmonella enterica serotype Pullorum. This disease primarily affects young chicks and can have significant consequences for poultry flocks. Here is an explanatory note on Bacillary White Diarrhea.

Indications: White diarrhea, Weakness, Poor growth, Loss of appetite, Chalky white excreta, poor feathering, enlarged liver and kidney with creamy caseous yolk sac.

Medicinal Management

- Acidum phosphoricum - Nervous exhaustion, Loss of vital fluid.
- Alumina - Sluggish GI functions, Feed contamination problems.
- Carbo vegetabilis - Cholera like symptoms, Venous congestion, weakness, loss of vital fluids.
- Iberis amara - White stool, Heart affections after influenza.
- Natrum sulph - Bio-chemic remedy for the supportive action. Helps to treat cold and flu. Cleansing of GI Tract.
- Mercurius corrosive - Rectal spasm, Albuminuria, white stool, gastric damages.
- Baptisia tinctoris - Diarrhea with acute fevers, Septic conditions.
- Cina - White colored stool, Fever, Loss of appetite.
- Calcarea Carb and Calcarea Phos – Chalky white, foamy diarrhea.
- Sulphur, Podophyllum and Ipecacuanha – Greenish brown diarrhea.
- Terminalia Arjuna – Severe diarrhea, Primary remedy for diarrhea.
- Arsenic album – Greenish diarrhea.

MYCOPLASMOSIS

Mycoplasma is a significant and persistent challenge in the poultry industry. Once a flock is infected, the infections tend to persist throughout the birds' lifespan. The primary mode of transmission is through vertical transmission, with the majority of birds acquiring the infection from infected parent stock. In contrast, horizontal transmission rates are comparatively lower.

A notable characteristic of Mycoplasma infections is the absence of cell walls in Mycoplasma species. This structural feature makes antibiotic treatments less effective compared to bacteria with cell walls, as many antibiotics target cell wall synthesis. As a result, managing Mycoplasma infections becomes more challenging.

In flocks that are free from Mycoplasma gallisepticum (MG) and Mycoplasma synoviae (MS), achieving optimal production becomes a complex task. The absence of cell walls in Mycoplasma makes them less susceptible to standard antibiotics, necessitating the use of bacteriostatic anti-mycoplasma drugs and vaccines.

While antibiotic treatments have limitations in Mycoplasma control, certain bacteriostatic drugs and vaccines have proven to be helpful to some extent. These measures aim to mitigate the impact of Mycoplasma infections, reduce clinical signs, and enhance overall flock health. The persistent nature of Mycoplasma infections underscores the importance of comprehensive management strategies, biosecurity practices, and ongoing monitoring to minimize the prevalence and impact of these challenging diseases in the poultry industry.

There are two main variants are present.

1) MG (Mycoplasma Gallisepticm)
2) MS (Mycoplams Synoviae).

Mycoplasma Gallisepticum (MG)

Mycoplasma gallisepticum (MG) is a causative agent responsible for inducing chronic respiratory diseases (CRD) in poultry. This bacterium has the capability to infect birds across all age groups, making it a significant concern in the poultry industry.

CRD is characterized by persistent and recurring respiratory symptoms in affected flocks. MG infections can lead to a range of respiratory issues, including coughing, sneezing, nasal discharge, and conjunctivitis. The chronic nature of the disease means that once a flock is infected, the respiratory problems may persist over an extended period.

The ability of MG to affect birds of all ages highlights its broad impact on poultry populations. In young chicks, MG infections can lead to slower growth rates and poor overall development. In laying hens, it may result in decreased egg production and poor egg quality. The ubiquitous nature of MG across different age groups emphasizes the need for comprehensive preventive measures, including biosecurity practices and vaccination strategies, to effectively manage and control the spread of Mycoplasma gallisepticum within poultry flocks.

Characteristics of Mycoplasma gallisepticum

- Mycoplasma gallisepticum **lacks a rigid cell wall,** making it more flexible and capable of assuming various shapes. This unique feature distinguishes it from typical bacteria.
- MG is primarily known as a respiratory pathogen in poultry. It infects the respiratory tract, leading to chronic respiratory diseases (CRD).

Clinical Signs and Symptoms: Infected birds exhibit respiratory signs such as coughing, sneezing, nasal discharge, and conjunctivitis. These symptoms contribute to the characteristic chronic respiratory disease. In laying hens, MG infections can lead to a drop in egg production and poor egg quality. MG can cause reproductive problems, including infertility, reduced hatchability, and the hatching of weak or infected chicks. The bacterium can affect birds of all ages, from chicks to mature layers and breeders, causing economic losses in the poultry industry.

Due to the absence of a cell wall, MG is less susceptible to many antibiotics. Treatment may involve the use of specific antibiotics, but success can be variable. Control measures often focus on prevention.

Transmission

- Vertical Transmission: MG can be transmitted vertically from infected breeder hens to their offspring through contaminated eggs.
- Horizontal Transmission: Direct contact between infected and susceptible birds, as well as contaminated fomites, contributes to horizontal transmission.

Medicinal Management

- Mycoplasma gallisepticum Nosode - Is a homeopathic nosode Stimulates the Immune system of birds and helps for selective phagocytosis.
- Curcuma longa - Anti-inflammatory, Anti-oxidant.
- Arsenic Album - Difficulty breathing, Opens beaks gasps for breath, Support to Respiratory cells, Low vital force.
- Adathoda vasica - Cough and cold.
- Ocimum Sanctum - Helps early recovery from respiratory health.
- Thuja occidentalis - Bronchitis, Expectorant.
- Naja Tripudians - Grasping at throat, with sense of choking.
- Belladonna - Anti-inflammatory, Sinusitis.
- Bryonia - Anti-inflammatory, Cold, Influenza, Low water intake.
- Arsenicum album - Anti Asthmatic, Saculitis.

Mycoplasma gallisepticum remains a significant challenge in the poultry industry, requiring a multifaceted approach for effective management. Regular monitoring, prompt diagnosis, and the implementation of preventive measures are crucial for minimizing the impact of MG on poultry flocks.

Mycoplasma Synoviae (MS)

Mycoplasma synoviae (MS) is a bacterium that plays a significant role in causing infectious synovitis, tendinitis, and various health issues in poultry, particularly in layer birds. Here's a descriptive note on the impact of MS and the associated clinical manifestations.

Characteristics of Mycoplasma synoviae

- Infectious Synovitis and Tendinitis: MS is a primary causative agent of infectious synovitis and tendinitis, leading to inflammation of the joints and tendons in affected birds.
- Leg Weakness and Lameness: The infection results in leg weakness and lameness, adversely affecting the mobility and overall well-being of the birds.
- Inflamed Joints: Joints become inflamed as a consequence of MS infection, contributing to the observed lameness and mobility issues.
- Pale Comb: Infected birds often display a pale comb, a visible sign of reduced vitality and overall health.
- Breast Biters: MS infection may lead to aggressive behaviors, such as breast biting, as birds experience discomfort and stress due to joint and tendon inflammation.
- Moderate Respiratory Tract Infections: Alongside joint and tendon issues, MS can cause moderate respiratory tract infections, further impacting the overall respiratory health of the affected birds.
- Egg Shell Abnormalities in Layer Birds: Layer birds infected with MS may experience egg shell abnormalities, leading to reduced egg quality and potential economic losses.

Transmission

- Horizontal Transmission: MS is primarily transmitted horizontally, spreading through direct contact between infected and susceptible birds or through contaminated fomites.
- Vertical Transmission: Transmission from infected breeder hens to their offspring can occur through contaminated eggs.

Medicinal Management

- Mycoplasma synoviae nososde - Prophylaxis care.
- Calacraea phos - Nutritive remedy for periosteum and bones.
- Calcarea carbonicum - Helps for bone diseases and blood.
- Hekla Lawa - Osteitis, Periostitis, Rachitis, Bone necrosis.
- Kali Hypo phosphoricum - Rickets, Osteitis, Respiratory illness.
- Acid phos - Helps to prevent periosteal inflammation, Neurosis, Fatigue and Stress.
- Chinium Sulph – Poly auricular remedy.
- Magnesium floratum – Localized inflammations, Muscular and neuralgic pains, Inflamed joints and tendons.
- Ruta graveolens - Pains, Tendinitis, Osteitis, Periostitis.

PROTOZOA

Protozoa infections in poultry, while less common than bacterial and viral infections, can still have significant impacts on the health and productivity of flocks.

1. **Coccidiosis** Coccidiosis stands as the most prevalent poultry disorder caused by protozoa, specifically Eimeria or Isospora species. This parasitic infection, characterized by the presence of coccidia, significantly impacts poultry health by invading the host and causing extensive damage to the entire intestinal system.

   Indications: The observed symptoms, including loss of appetite, weight loss, low feed conversion ratio, bloody diarrhea, dehydration, dropping feathers, and acute death, collectively indicate a complex set of health issues in poultry.

Clinical Impact

- Intestinal System Damage: Coccidia parasites specifically target the intestinal tract, causing damage to the mucosal lining and epithelial cells.
- Enteritis: The invasion of coccidia leads to enteritis, characterized by inflammation of the intestines, resulting in diarrhea.
- Dehydration: Severe cases can lead to dehydration due to the loss of fluids through diarrhea, affecting the overall well-being of the birds.

Transmission

- Fecal-Oral Route: The life cycle of coccidia involves shedding of oocysts in the feces of infected birds. The ingestion of contamination.

Medicinal Management

- Merc cor - Birds bloody drooping.
- Nux vomica - Lack of appetite, GI disturbances.
- Chelidonium - Pale comb, inflamed liver.
- Sulphur - pale comb, fortify the action of other remedy.
- Merc sol - Bloody, slimy diarrhea, cecal cocci.
- Ipecacuanha - Hemorrhages, cocci in birds, vomiting, drooping.
- Filix Mas – Tape worm infestations, Helps expels the worms from body.
- Chenopodium – Anti worming property, Especially Hook works and Round worms.
- Chimaphilia maculata – Worm fever.
- Cina – Loss of appetite, Weakness, Worm infestations.
- Passiflora incarnate – Extreme fatigue, Poor nutrition.
- Scilla maritima – Gut and intestinal health, recorrect the worm infestation complaints.
- Swertia chirata – Worm complaints, Fever, Digestive disorders.

OTHER PROFICIENCY TOPICS

1. LIVER HEALTH SOLUTIONS

The liver is a vital and the largest organ in chickens, playing a crucial role in maintaining overall health and metabolic functions. Unlike humans, avian livers have two lobes, each containing thousands of hepatic cells. The major functions of the avian liver are akin to those in humans, encompassing metabolism of proteins, carbohydrates, and fats, storage of nutrients, detoxification, digestion, synthesis of essential molecules, and regulation of lipogenesis and lipolysis.

Avian Liver Structure and Functions:

- Organ Size and Structure: The liver in birds, comprising two lobes, consists of numerous hepatic cells arranged in lobes. This intricate structure facilitates the organ's multifaceted functions.
- Metabolic Functions: Similar to humans, avian livers are involved in metabolic processes, including the breakdown and utilization of proteins, carbohydrates, and fats.
- Storage of Nutrients: The liver serves as a storage reservoir for essential nutrients, ensuring a steady supply during periods of high demand or scarcity.
- Detoxification: Detoxification processes in the liver involve the neutralization and elimination of harmful substances, safeguarding the bird from toxins.
- Digestion: The liver contributes to digestion by producing bile, a substance crucial for the emulsification and absorption of fats in the digestive system.

- Synthesis of Essential Molecules: The synthesis of proteins, enzymes, and other vital molecules occurs in the liver, supporting various physiological functions.
- Regulation of Lipogenesis and Lipolysis: The liver plays a role in the regulation of lipid metabolism, controlling the synthesis and breakdown of fats.
- Maintaining optimal liver health is crucial for the overall performance of birds in poultry farming, influencing growth, reproduction, and disease resistance.

Liver disorders in poultry can arise from a variety of factors, both infectious and noninfectious, leading to the destruction of hepatic cells and disruption of normal liver functions. One prevalent liver disorder in poultry is Avian Hepatitis, primarily caused by the Avian Hepatitis E virus (aHEV), which shares genetic similarities with the Human Hepatitis E Virus. Additionally, inactivated vaccines, mycotoxins, and aflatoxins are identified as noninfectious factors that can contribute to liver damage.

Common Challenges: Mycotoxins, often found in contaminated feed, pose a significant challenge to avian liver health, potentially impairing its functions.

Clinical Consequences

- Hepatic Cell Destruction: Liver disorders result in the destruction of hepatic cells, compromising the organ's structural integrity and functionality.
- Disruption of Normal Liver Functions: Normal liver functions, including metabolism, detoxification, and synthesis, are disrupted, leading to systemic consequences.

Indicators of Liver Health: The color of the liver serves as an indicator of health status. At 8 to 10 weeks, the liver exhibits a yellowish color due to yolk content absorption, gradually transitioning to brown thereafter.

Treatment Protocols: Implementing suitable treatment protocols for liver-related issues, including addressing mycotoxin contamination, is essential.

Supplementary Solutions: Providing supplementary solutions, such as liver-supporting supplements, aids in maintaining optimal liver function.

The avian liver, with its central role in metabolic and physiological functions, is indispensable for the well-being and performance of poultry. Monitoring liver health, addressing challenges like mycotoxin contamination, and implementing appropriate treatment and supplementation protocols are vital steps toward ensuring the overall productivity and success of poultry farming operations.

Many infectious and noninfectious factors are responsible for liver disorders, it will destruct the hepatic cells and interrupt the normal liver functions. Avian Hepatitis is the common poultry liver disorder infected by Avian hepatitis E virus (aHEV), genetically similar like Human Hepatitis E Virus. Some of inactivated vaccines, Mycotoxins and aflatoxin are also responsible for liver damage.

Medicinal Management

- Nux vomica - Polychrest remedy, Hepatitis.
- Silibum marianum – Action over liver portal system, Dropsy, Hepatitis.
- Lycopodium - Hepatitis, Anti stress, Malnutrition, Ascites, Simultaneous action over the liver and kidney.
- Ceaonanthus - Stimulate hepatic filtration, Acted over liver and spleen.
- Chelidonium - Enzymatic actions, Anti tumour & genotoxic activity. Prominent liver remedy. Hepatitis, Bile obstructions.
- Myrica cerifera - Stimulate hepatic filtration, jaundice, acted over hepatic mucous membrane.
- Grindelia Robusta - Anti oxidant activity, detoxification. Splenic symptoms, Hyperemia.
- Kalmegh - Antioxidant and Anti-inflammatory, increase bile secretions, laxative.
- Berberis aristata - Hepatomegaly, Hepato toxicity, Spleenomegaly.
- Terminalia chebula - Increase bile secretions.
- Cardu marianus - Anti oxidant, Marked action over the liver.

- Taraxacum officinalis - Helps clear to liver obstruction and remove toxins from the Blood.

Liver disorders, whether infectious or noninfectious, significantly affect the health and productivity of poultry. Monitoring, timely diagnosis, and the implementation of preventive measures are crucial for sustaining the overall performance of poultry farming operations. Understanding the various factors contributing to liver disorders aids in the development of comprehensive management strategies for maintaining optimal liver health in poultry flocks.

2. KIDNEY HEALTH SOLUTIONS

The kidneys serve as the excretory system in birds, with each bird having two kidneys. Their primary function is to filter waste and toxins from the blood. Unlike humans, fowl do not possess a bladder. Instead, the kidneys are connected to the ureters, and these open into the cloaca. The urine then moves from the cloaca to the large intestine through reverse peristalsis movement. The urine, appearing thick and whitish, is expelled along with the stool. Kidney dysfunctions in poultry can result from various factors, including nephrotoxins, the nephrogenic form of the Infectious Bronchitis (IB) virus, and a high-protein diet. These dysfunctions can lead to the deposition of uric acid and pose significant challenges in the form of nephrotoxicities for poultry birds.

Kidney Function in Birds

- Excretory System: The kidneys play a crucial role as the excretory system, filtering waste and toxins from the blood.

- Absence of Bladder: Unlike humans, fowl lack a bladder. Instead, urine is transported from the kidneys to the cloaca via ureters.
- Connection to Cloaca: The ureters connect to the cloaca, and urine is expelled from the cloaca, along with feces, through reverse peristalsis movement.
- Uric Acid Deposition: Birds excrete uric acid, which appears as a thick, whitish substance, along with feces.

Causes of Kidney Dysfunctions

- Nephrotoxins: Exposure to nephrotoxic substances can lead to kidney dysfunction in poultry.
- Nephrogenic IB Virus: The nephrogenic form of the Infectious Bronchitis (IB) virus is a causative factor for kidney issues in birds.
- High Protein Diet: A diet excessively high in protein may contribute to kidney dysfunctions in poultry.

Consequences of Kidney Dysfunctions

- Uric Acid Deposition: Kidney dysfunctions can result in the deposition of uric acid, leading to alterations in urine composition.
- Nephrotoxicities: The impaired function of the kidneys can result in nephrotoxicities, presenting a major challenge for poultry health. Nephrotoxicities pose significant challenges as they impact the kidneys' ability to regulate fluid and electrolyte balance.

Medicinal Management

- Lycopodium - Polychrest Remedy, Anti Inflammatory, helps to improve all kidney and Liver functions. Chronic gout with chalky deposit in the joints, helps prevent uric acid deposition in the body.
- Berberis vulgaris - Cystitis, Infections in kidney, helps to recover impairment of kidney, Improve the kidney functions and induce to excrete waste products.
- Benzoicum acidum - A remedy of great antiseptic powers. Inflammation.
- Uva ursi - Helps in the elimination of uric acid from the body. hive-like eruptions in the joints.
- Copaiva Officinalis - Acted powerfully over the urinary tract mucous membrane.
- Fuchsinum - Degeneration of kidney.
- Cantharis - Liquidation of uric acid crystals and urates.
- Apocyanum - Accelerate purifying activity of nephrons.
- Chimaphilia umbellata - Improve kidney filtration activity, acted over kidneys and genito urinary tract.
- Arbutinum - Urinary antiseptic and diuretic.

3. REPRODUCTIVE HEALTH SOLUTIONS

The avian reproductive system operates on a heterosexual basis, with male birds producing sperm from their testes, while female birds contribute ovum (yolk) produced by the ovary. The female reproductive anatomy comprises two main components: the ovary and the oviduct. Ovum development occurs in the ovary, and upon maturation, it is released into the oviduct. After fertilization, the oviduct glands secrete albumin (egg white), and the shell is formed, resulting in the complete egg. The entire process of egg formation takes approximately 26 hours from the matured yolk.

Avian Reproductive System Components

- Testes (Male): Male birds produce sperm from the testes.
- Ovary (Female): The ovary is responsible for the development of ovum (yolk) in female birds.
- Oviduct (Female): The oviduct is a crucial part of the female reproductive system where egg formation takes place, including the secretion of albumin and shell formation.
- Egg Formation Process:
  Ovum Development - Ovum matures in the ovary.
  Release into Oviduct - Matured ovum is released into the oviduct.
  Fertilization - Fertilization occurs, initiating the process of egg formation.
  Albumin Secretion - Oviduct glands secrete albumin (egg white).
  Shell Formation - The shell is formed, completing the egg.

The entire process, from the matured yolk to the formation of a complete egg, takes approximately 26 hours. Once an egg is laid, the hen ovulates a new yolk, continuing the reproductive cycle.

Reproductive Lifespan and Productivity

- Reproductive Lifespan: Flocks have a reproductive lifespan of 3-4 years, with the quantity and quality of egg production potentially decreasing each year.
- Seasonal Influence: Maximum egg production is often achieved during the summer seasons.

Reproductive health is crucial for poultry, and ensuring the well-being of the flock involves providing supplementary nutrition and implementing treatment management strategies. This is essential for maintaining and enhancing the productivity of the birds.

Medicinal Management

- Acid Phos - Hair loss in face and genitals, Promote fertility.
- Withenia Somniferous - Improves the male vigor. Spermatorrhoea.
- Aurum metallicum - Helps to produce more quantity of semen.
- Staphysagriya - improves the male vigor.
- Damiana - Helps to stimulate the testes to secrete testosterone.
- Agnus Castus - Hormonal activity.
- Makardwaja – Aphrodisiac.
- Thuja occidentalis - Miasmatic remedy, Improve viability of sperm.
- Medorrhinum - Miasmatic remedy.
- Calcarea (Calcarea phos, sulph, carb) - Malabsorption Calcium, Assimilatory deffects in calcium metabolism, Increases the tonicity of the uterine wall, releasing stable calcium for better egg.
- Cimicifuga racemose - For ovarian irritation.

- Natrum carbonicum - For the effective retention of sperm.
- Pulsatilla nigricans - Synchronize the ovulation.
- Natrum muriaticum - Improve the quality of mucus, helps sperm preservation.
- Folliculinum - Stimulate ovulation. Helps to stimulate FSH and LH.
- Muira pauma – Aphrodisiac.
- Conium maculatum – Glandular enhancement.
- Damiana – Sexual Neurasthenia.

Understanding the intricacies of the avian reproductive system, including the processes of ovum development, fertilization, and egg formation, is essential for effective poultry management. Regular monitoring, proper nutrition, and attentive care contribute to maintaining reproductive health and sustaining optimal productivity in poultry flocks.

4. GROWTH PROMOTERS

The discovery of antibiotics has been a transformative development in controlling infectious diseases in both humans and animals, significantly contributing to the improvement of the economic status of the food animal production industry. In animal agriculture, antibiotics have been utilized as growth-promoting agents, commonly referred to as Antibiotic Growth Promoters (AGP). However, the non-therapeutic use of antibiotics, particularly in subtherapeutic doses for growth promotion, has raised concerns related to antibiotic resistance, environmental impact, public health risks, and food chain safety. In response to these concerns, there has been a shift towards alternative approaches, leading to the emergence of organic farming and the use of Natural Growth Promoters (NGP).

Antibiotics in Animal Agriculture: Antibiotics have played a crucial role in controlling and preventing infectious diseases in both humans and animals, contributing to the overall health of food-producing animals. The use of antibiotics in animal agriculture has improved the economic viability of food animal production by reducing disease-related losses and promoting growth.

Antibiotic Growth Promoters (AGP): Antibiotic Growth Promoters have been employed in animal farming to enhance growth rates and improve feed efficiency, leading to increased weight gain in animals.

Concerns Associated with AGP: Non-therapeutic use of antibiotics for growth promotion has raised concerns, including the development of antibiotic resistance, potential environmental consequences, risks to public health, and safety concerns in the food chain.

Alternative Approaches: Organic Farming and NGP: Organic farming emphasizes natural and sustainable practices, limiting the use of synthetic chemicals, including antibiotics. It aims to promote animal health through holistic and preventive measures.

Natural Growth Promoters (NGP): NGPs are alternatives to traditional AGPs, encompassing natural substances, plant extracts, probiotics, prebiotics, and other nutritional additives that promote growth and enhance animal health without the use of antibiotics.

Growth promoters, whether in the form of traditional AGPs, NGPs, or through organic farming practices, play a pivotal role in enhancing weight gain and promoting the overall health and productivity of poultry and other food-producing animals. Homeopathy, a form of alternative medicine, involves the use of highly diluted substances derived from plants, minerals, or animals to stimulate the body's natural healing processes. In recent years, there has been interest in exploring the potential of homeopathy as a natural growth promoter (NGP) in animal agriculture, including poultry farming.

Medicinal Management

- Medicago Sativa - Enhance appetite, Promote weight gain. Helps to increase Increase digestive secretions an HDL.
- Withenia Somnifera - improve the permeability of epithelial tissue of intestine.
- Calcarea Carbonica Oatrearum - Impaired Nutrition.
- Avena Sativa - Gut health promoter, Promote Fat, Proteins metabolism, enhance feed conversion ratio, intestinal motility helping in digestion and assimilation.
- Alaninum-D - Alanine is an α-amino acid that is used in the bio synthesis, Used as growth factor.
- Argininum – Stimulate growth hormones, Essential for Infants (Alpha Amino Acids used for the Bio synthesis of Proteins).
- Iodium - Rapid metabolizer and lack of flesh.
- Allium sativa - Lipid digestion, Anti-microbial.
- Chamommile - Promote protease and enzymatic activity.
- Carrica papaya - immune-stimulating, Helps for the Breaks down of proteins.
- Curcuma long - Anti-inflammatory and Antioxidant.

5. IMMUNE MODULATOR

Immune modulators are substances or agents that aid in the activation, enhancement, or restoration of normal immune functions in the context of a compromised or deranged immune system. In poultry birds, maintaining a balanced and functional immune system is crucial for overall health and disease resistance. Immune system derangement in poultry can result in a range of negative consequences, including frequent infections, an increased risk of secondary infections, diminished response to drug therapies and vaccines, and heightened pathogenicity.'

In the current landscape of poultry farming, there is a notable emphasis on chemotherapy and diseases-based treatment protocols. Despite these efforts, the poultry industry continues to grapple with challenges such as multi-infections, the emergence and re-emergence of diseases, the presence of chemical residues in meat, and concerns related to public health and environmental safety. In response to these challenges, immune therapy has emerged as a potential strategy to address some of the issues facing the poultry industry.

Importance of Immune Therapy in Poultry

- Complementing Traditional Approaches: Immune therapy serves as a complementary approach to traditional chemotherapy and treatment protocols. Instead of solely targeting specific pathogens, immune therapy focuses on enhancing the overall immune system of poultry.
- Multi-Infections and Disease Challenges: Poultry often faces the complexity of multi-infections and the constant challenge of diseases. Immune therapy

aims to bolster the birds' natural defense mechanisms, making them more resilient to a variety of pathogens.

- Emergence and Re-emergence of Diseases: The dynamic nature of diseases, including their emergence and re-emergence, necessitates a proactive approach. Immune therapy provides a means to strengthen the birds' immune responses, potentially reducing the impact of emerging diseases.
- Chemical Residues and Food Safety: Concerns about chemical residues in meat have heightened awareness regarding food safety. By focusing on immune therapy, there is an opportunity to reduce reliance on certain chemical treatments and promote a more natural and sustainable approach to poultry health.
- Public Health and Environmental Safety: Immune therapy aligns with concerns about public health and environmental safety. By minimizing the use of certain chemicals and antibiotics, it contributes to a safer and more sustainable poultry production system.

Risk Factors of Poultry Immunity: Poultry immunity, crucial for the overall health and disease resistance of birds, can be influenced by various risk factors. Understanding and mitigating these factors is essential for maintaining robust immunity in poultry flocks.

1. **Infections:**
    - Viral Infections: Viruses pose a significant threat to poultry immunity, leading to diseases such as

Newcastle disease, avian influenza, and infectious bronchitis.

- Mycoplasma Infections: Mycoplasma infections, including Mycoplasma gallisepticum and Mycoplasma synoviae, can compromise the respiratory and reproductive systems in poultry.
- Coccidiosis: Coccidiosis, caused by protozoan parasites, is a common poultry disease affecting the intestinal tract and impairing immune function.
- E. coli Infections: Infections by Escherichia coli (E. coli) can result in respiratory and systemic diseases, impacting the immune response in poultry.

2. **Mycotoxins:**
   - Aflatoxins: Aflatoxins, produced by certain molds, can contaminate feed and impair poultry immunity, leading to various health issues.
   - Trichothecenes, Ochratoxins, Rubratoxins, Patulin, Citrinin, etc.: Other mycotoxins, including trichothecenes, ochratoxins, rubratoxins, patulin, and citrinin, present in contaminated feed, pose risks to immune function.

3. **Inadequate Nutrition:**
   - Nutritional Deficiencies: Inadequate nutrition, marked by deficiencies in essential vitamins, minerals, and amino acids, can compromise the immune system's ability to function optimally.

4. **Non-Therapeutic Chemotherapy:**
   - Antibiotic Misuse: Non-therapeutic use of antibiotics, including suboptimal dosages or unnecessary administration, can contribute to antibiotic resistance and weaken the immune response.

5. **Stress:**
   - Environmental Stress: Environmental stressors such as high stocking density, poor ventilation, and extreme temperatures can induce stress, negatively impacting the immune system.
   - Transportation Stress: The stress associated with transportation can weaken the immune response, making birds more susceptible to diseases upon arrival.
6. **Genomic Mutations:**
   - Genetic Factors: Genomic mutations and genetic predispositions can influence the efficacy of the immune system, potentially rendering birds more susceptible to infections.

Comparison between Immune System of Human and Chicken

IMMUNE SYSTEM	SIMILARITIES	CHICKEN	HUMAN
LYMPHATICS SYSTEM	Thymus, Tonsils Spleen, Basophils Eosinophils,	Bursa of Fabricius, Heterophils Harderian Glands	Bone Marrow Neutrophils Lymph Nodes.
ANTIGEN PRESENTING CELLS	Dentric Cells Macrophages	Unknown Location	Lymph Nodes
ANTIBODY	IgM, IgA	IgY	IgG, IgE, IgD

Credits: www.researchgate.net/profile/Zuzana-Macek-Jilkova-2/publication.

Mechanisms of Immune Therapy

1. Immunostimulant: Immune therapy involves the stimulation of the bird's immune system. This can be achieved through various means, including the use of immunomodulators, vaccines, and natural substances that enhance immune responses.
2. Boosting Natural Defenses: The goal of immune therapy is to boost the natural defenses of poultry, making them more adept at recognizing and neutralizing pathogens.
3. Adaptive Responses: Immune therapy supports the development of adaptive immune responses, allowing birds to mount effective defenses upon exposure to specific pathogens.

Methods to Enhance Poultry Immunity

1. Adopt Antibiotic-Free Feeding Strategies: Transitioning to antibiotic-free feeding strategies is a key approach to promote poultry immunity. This helps in reducing the reliance on antibiotics and encourages the development of a robust and natural immune system.
2. Set Innovative Gut Performance Management Solutions: Implementing innovative solutions for gut performance management is crucial. This includes strategies to maintain gut health, optimize nutrient absorption, and foster a balanced microbiome, all of which contribute to enhanced immunity.
3. Enhance Maternal Immunity: Enhancing maternal immunity is fundamental for providing newborn chicks with a strong foundation of immune

protection. This involves nutritional interventions for breeding hens to pass on vital antibodies and immune factors to their offspring.

4. Maintain Normal Intestinal Microbiota: Ensuring the maintenance of normal intestinal microbiota is essential for supporting immune function. Strategies such as probiotic supplementation can aid in preserving a healthy balance of beneficial bacteria in the gut.
5. Stimulate Immune Response: Actively stimulating the immune response is a proactive measure. This can be achieved through the use of immunomodulators, vaccines, and other agents that enhance the recognition and response of the immune system to pathogens.
6. Produce Anti-microbial and Anti-viral Substances: Implementing measures that encourage the production of anti-microbial and anti-viral substances within the poultry system contributes to the defense against pathogens. This may involve dietary supplements or natural additives with such properties.
7. Improve Hormonal and Enzymatic Activity: Enhancing hormonal and enzymatic activity is vital for the proper functioning of various physiological processes, including immune responses. Optimal hormonal balance and enzyme activity support overall health and immune system efficiency.

8. Promote Antioxidant Index: Promoting a high antioxidant index is crucial for mitigating oxidative stress, which can compromise immune function. Including antioxidant-rich components in the diet helps neutralize free radicals and support a healthier immune system.

Medicinal Managements:

Homeopathic medications play a role in modulating the immune system of birds, exhibiting both normal and biologically induced forms. This term encompasses the concept of homeostasis within the immune system, wherein the system self-regulates.

- Emblica Officinalis - Anemia, Gastric disturbances, Immune Stimulants, Heat Stress.
- Zingiber officinalis - Improve the permeability of epithelial tissue of intestine, Antibacterial, Promote kidney functions.
- Beta vulgaris - Prevent chronic catarrhal conditions, provide good yield.
- Arsenicum album - Higher viral load with lower cd4 count, Hypochondriac anxiety, Protect MT4 cell viability against toxicity, Acted over leukocytes.
- Avena Sativa - Improve nutritional functioning.
- Carica papaya - can mediate a Th1 type shift in human immune system. Helps to increase WBS and Platelet count.
- Thymus vulgaris – Control T-lymphocytes
- Lecithinum - Helps in the maintenance of Hemoglobin and health of brain, Increases the number of Red Corpuscles (RBC) and amount of Hemoglobin.

- Withenia sominifera – Enhance immunity. Responsible for hormonal activities, Adaptogen.
- Ginseng - improve the permeability of epithelial tissue of intestine. Energizer.
- Oscimum sanctum – Immune modulator, Antioxidant.
- Alfa alfa - Malnutrition, appetizer.
- Malandrinum & Tuja - Preventive bad effects of vaccines.
- Muringa oleifera - Neutrophil adhesion, DTH reactions.

These methods collectively contribute to the development of a robust immune system in poultry, promoting overall health and resilience to diseases. Adopting a holistic approach that considers various aspects of nutrition, gut health, and immune stimulation is key to achieving sustained improvements in poultry immunity.

Bio-Markers for Poultry Immunity

Biomarkers in poultry immunity are measurable indicators that provide valuable information about the state and effectiveness of the immune system in birds. These markers aid in assessing the health, disease resistance, and overall immune competence of poultry flocks.

- Immune Organ Index (g/Kg): Weight of immune organs (g) / Live body weight (Kg). This index quantifies the relative size and development of immune organs, providing insight into the overall health and functionality of the immune system.
- PBMC (Peripheral Blood Mononuclear Cell) Isolation & Proliferation: Isolation and assessment of PBMCs allow for the evaluation of the immune

system's responsiveness and ability to mount an immune response.

- Blood Parameters (Hb, WBC, RBC, pH, Lipid Profile): Various blood parameters, including Hemoglobin (Hb), White Blood Cells (WBC), Red Blood Cells (RBC), pH, and Lipid Profile, offer comprehensive information about the physiological status and immune competence of the birds.
- Liver Function Test: Evaluates markers of liver health, providing insights into the organ's metabolic functions and its impact on overall immunity.
- Kidney Function Test: Assesses the renal function to understand the excretory system's role in maintaining homeostasis and its potential impact on immune responses.
- Histopathology of Immune Organs (Liver, Bursa, Thymus): Microscopic examination of immune organs allows for the identification of structural changes, inflammation, or abnormalities, indicating potential immune system challenges.
- Determination of T-Cell Subsets, B-Cells, and Monocytes/Macrophages in Peripheral Mononuclear Cells (PBMCs) by Flow Cytometry: Flow cytometry enables the precise quantification of different immune cell populations, providing a detailed analysis of the cellular components of the immune system.
- Spectrometric Determination of Serum Lysozyme Activity: Measures the lysozyme activity in the serum, an enzyme with antimicrobial properties, indicating the bird's ability to combat bacterial infections.

- Determination of Serum Cytokines, Immunoglobulin, and Ileal sIgA Levels by ELISA: Enzyme-Linked Immunosorbent Assay (ELISA) quantifies various immune markers, including cytokines, immunoglobulins, and secretory Immunoglobulin A (sIgA), reflecting the immune response at the molecular level.
- Serum Bacterial Activity: Assesses the serum's ability to exhibit antimicrobial activity, providing an indication of the bird's resistance to bacterial infections.
- Antibody Titre Value in Blood: Measures the concentration of specific antibodies in the blood, indicating the strength of the immune response to particular antigens.
- Immunoglobulin Analysis (IgM, IgA, IgG): Differentiates and quantifies specific immunoglobulin classes, providing a nuanced understanding of the humoral immune response.
- Hormonal Assay (Thyroid, TSH, GH, ACTH, Testosterone): Assesses hormonal levels related to the endocrine system, which plays a crucial role in modulating immune responses and overall health.

These comprehensive bio-markers collectively offer a detailed and multifaceted assessment of poultry immunity, aiding in the identification of potential challenges and the development of targeted management strategies for optimal immune function.

6. **BEHAVIOURAL DISORDER SOLUTIONS**

CANNIBALISM: Consuming all or part of another individual of the same species as food. Seen domestic egg laying species. Mal Nutritional defiance – Sulphur containing proteins (Methionine). It is a main frame work of feather. Due to Stress, Overcrowding, Heat & Hereditary. As per the symptom's similarities.

1. **Ignatia-** Nervous temperament, Contradictory behavior.
2. **Sulphur**

7. **ENVIRONMENTAL FACTORS RELATED SOLUTIONS**

Environmental factors play a crucial role in the health and well-being of poultry. Various conditions and stressors within the environment can contribute to disorders and impact the overall health of the flock.

- **Heat Stress:** Heat stress occurs when poultry are exposed to high temperatures beyond their comfort range. This environmental challenge can lead to reduced feed intake, increased water consumption, panting, and behavioral changes. Severe cases may result in heat exhaustion or even death. Proper ventilation, shading, and cooling methods are essential to prevent and manage heat stress in poultry.

Medicinal Management

- **Natrum mur:** Natrum Mur is indicated for normalizing the body's metabolism by regulating electrolyte balance mechanisms. In the context of heat stress, it helps maintain the body's fluid balance and supports overall metabolic functions. This remedy is beneficial for individuals experiencing imbalances due to excessive heat.

- **Natrum carb:** Natrum Carb is used to counteract the adverse effects of summer heat and sunstroke. It addresses indigestion problems arising from excessive heat exposure. This remedy is particularly useful for individuals who may experience digestive disturbances during hot weather.
- **Mentha Piperita:** Mentha Piperita, derived from peppermint, stimulates the cold-perceiving nerves. It has marked action on the respiratory organs and skin. This remedy can be beneficial for providing a cooling effect and relieving discomfort associated with heat stress. It may also address respiratory issues exacerbated by heat.
- **Glonine:** Glonine is indicated for hyperemia of the brain resulting from excessive exposure to both cold and heat, including conditions like sunstroke. It helps alleviate symptoms related to cerebral congestion, providing relief from throbbing headaches and other manifestations of heat stress.
- **Gelsemium:** Gelsemium is valuable in cases of dehydration, prostration, and whitish watery diarrhea, which can occur during heat stress. It addresses symptoms of weakness and exhaustion, making it a suitable remedy for conditions where there is a loss of fluids due to excessive heat.
- **Sulphur:** Sulphur is known for its efficacy in cases of acute stress and sensitivity to atmospheric changes. In individuals with warm-blooded

constitutions, Sulphur addresses complaints arising from warmth in general. It may help restore balance in those experiencing stress-related symptoms exacerbated by heat.

- **Calendula:** Calendula is beneficial for managing heat stress and post-traumatic edema. It possesses healing properties that can assist in reducing inflammation and promoting recovery from the effects of heat stress. Calendula is often used externally for its wound-healing properties.
- **Handling & Transportation Stress:** Improper handling during catching, transportation, and rehousing can induce stress in poultry. Stress during these processes may result in injuries, reduced feed intake, and increased susceptibility to diseases. Careful and gentle handling practices, as well as proper transportation protocols, are crucial to minimize stress-related health issues.

Medicinal Management

- Nux vomica: Nux Vomica is well-suited for individuals who exhibit nervousness and irritability. In the context of handling and transportation stress, it addresses symptoms related to heightened sensitivity, restlessness, and irritability. Nux Vomica can be beneficial for calming the nervous system and reducing stress associated with these situations.
- Arnica montana: Arnica Montana is known for its effectiveness in managing physical exhaustion and stress. In the context of handling and transportation, where birds may experience physical exertion and

stress, Arnica helps alleviate soreness, bruising, and overall physical discomfort. It supports recovery from the physical strain associated with transportation.

- Five phos: Five Phos is a tissue salt that plays a role in maintaining minerals and electrolyte balance. During handling and transportation, birds may experience changes in their electrolyte balance. Five Phos helps in restoring and maintaining proper mineral balance, thereby supporting the overall well-being of poultry during stressful situations.
- **Traumatic Stress:** Traumatic stress can result from physical injuries, such as pecking, fighting, or accidental injuries. It may lead to pain, inflammation, and behavioral changes. Implementing preventive measures, providing suitable housing, and monitoring bird interactions can help reduce the risk of traumatic stress.

Medicinal Management

- **Thuja:** Thuja is indicated for addressing the adverse effects associated with vaccination. It is particularly useful in cases where birds exhibit symptoms or reactions following vaccination. Thuja helps in mitigating the negative effects and supporting the overall well-being of the birds after vaccination.
- **Arnica Montana:** Arnica is known for its effectiveness in managing bruised injuries. In the context of vaccination, where injections may cause localized bruising or soreness, Arnica helps alleviate these symptoms. It is beneficial for reducing pain

and promoting recovery after the physical stress of vaccination.

- **Hypericum:** Hypericum is indicated for hard injuries and nerve injuries. In the context of vaccination, where there may be discomfort or nerve-related symptoms, Hypericum provides relief. It is particularly useful in addressing pain or sensitivity associated with nerve injuries caused by injections.
- **Vaccinum, Tuja & Malandrinum:**
This combination is used for the prevention of smallpox and to counteract the potential adverse effects of vaccines. Vaccinum, Thuja, and Malandrinum together create a homeopathic prophylactic approach, helping to minimize the negative impacts of vaccination and support the birds' immune responses.
- **Cold Stress:** Cold stress occurs in colder climates or during extreme weather conditions. Poultry exposed to low temperatures may experience reduced egg production, slower growth, and increased susceptibility to respiratory infections. Adequate insulation, heating, and provision of warm bedding are necessary to mitigate cold stress.
- **Overcrowding:** Overcrowding in poultry houses can lead to stress, aggression, and the spread of diseases. Birds may exhibit aggressive behaviors such as cannibalism, feather pecking, and reduced egg production. Proper housing design and management practices, including optimal stocking density, are crucial to prevent overcrowding-related disorders.

In conclusion, a holistic approach to poultry management involves proactive measures to create a conducive environment that minimizes stressors. Regular monitoring, prompt intervention, and continuous improvement in housing and management practices contribute to the overall health, productivity, and welfare of poultry flocks. A well-managed environment ensures that birds can express their natural behaviors and thrive in a stress-free setting.

HOMEOPATHIC SOLUTIONS FOR VETERINARY PRACTICE

Homeopathic veterinary solutions represent a holistic and natural approach to animal health and well-being. Derived from the principles of homeopathy, these solutions aim to address the underlying causes of health issues in animals, promoting balance and supporting the body's innate healing abilities.

Key Components of Homeopathic Veterinary Solutions

- Individualized Treatment: Homeopathy recognizes the unique constitution of each animal. Veterinary homeopaths assess not only the specific symptoms but also the animal's overall temperament, behavior, and environmental factors to tailor individualized treatment plans.
- Natural Healing Principles: Homeopathic remedies are prepared from natural sources, such as plants, minerals, and animal substances. These highly diluted substances stimulate the body's vital force, encouraging self-healing without causing harm or side effects.
- Holistic Approach: Homeopathic veterinary care considers the whole animal, addressing physical, mental, and emotional aspects of health. This holistic approach aims to restore balance and vitality in the animal's life.
- Prevention and Wellness: Homeopathy can be used preventively to maintain overall health and prevent the development of chronic conditions. It emphasizes wellness and vitality, supporting the animal's resilience against diseases.

- Complementary to Conventional Care: Homeopathic veterinary solutions can be used alongside conventional veterinary treatments. Integrative approaches allow for a comprehensive and synergistic approach to animal health, combining the strengths of both systems.
- Minimal Side Effects:Due to the highly diluted nature of homeopathic remedies, they are generally well-tolerated by animals. This makes homeopathic solutions a safe option with minimal risk of adverse effects.
- Broad Range of Applications: Homeopathy can address a wide range of health issues in animals, including acute conditions (such as injuries and infections) and chronic diseases. It is suitable for various species, including dogs, cats, horses, livestock, and exotic animals.
- Environmental and Ethical Considerations: Homeopathic remedies are often prepared using sustainable and ethical practices. This aligns with a growing awareness of the impact of conventional practices on the environment and animal welfare.

Benefits of Homeopathic Veterinary Solutions

- Gentle and Non-Invasive: Homeopathy provides a non-invasive and gentle approach to treating animals, making it suitable for animals of all ages and conditions.
- Reduced Resistance: Homeopathic remedies work with the body's natural processes, potentially reducing the development of resistance seen with some conventional medications.
- Support for Chronic Conditions: Homeopathy can be particularly beneficial in managing chronic conditions where conventional treatments may offer limited relief.

QUICK REMEDY PROFILE

Understanding the characteristics and applications of different remedies is essential in homeopathic medicine. A quick remedy profile serves as a concise reference guide, providing key information about individual remedies. This introduction aims to highlight the importance of remedy profiles in homeopathy.

SL. NO	REMEDY	INDICATIONS
1	Acidum Phos	Poor feathering, Weakness
2	Aconitum napellus	Anxiety, Cough & Cold, Fever Acute illness, Anti-Viral Influenza, Hyper sensitive.
3	Agnus castus	Helps to stimulates testosterone.
4	Allium Sativa	Anti-Viral, Lower blood lipids.
5	Arnica montana	Injuries, Bruising, Hemorrhages, Stress (Traumatic, Handling and Transportation).
6	Arsenicum album	Respiratory illness, Ailments Cold, General weakness, Polychrest, Anti-Viral.
7	Aspidosperma	Pneumatic center simulations.
8	Aurum met	Improve viability of sperm.
9	Aviaire	Action over lung, Improve appetite.
10	Azadirachta indica	Antioxidant and Antiseptic.
11	Bacillus substile	Gut health.
12	Belladonna	Anti-inflammatory, Fever, Fatigue, Air sickness, Prevent damage of CNS. Analgesic.
13	Borax	Ulcers, Copper sulfate oral lesions.
14	Calcarea	Increase tonicity of uterine wall.
15	Cal Phos	Egg, Bone & Skeletal Health
16	Causticum	Horny Cutaneous skin lesions during Fowl pox.

17	Cicuta Virosa	Renikhet diseases, Torticollis and Spine deformity.
18	Cimicifuga	Oophoritis, Ovarian Irritations Yolk sac infections.
19	Cina	De wormer (Filix Mas) White colored stool.
20	Colchicum	Gout.
21	Echinacea	Blood purifier, immune modulator, Antibacterial.
22	Ferrum Met	Improve Hemoglobin.
23	Ferrum Phos	Antipyretic and Acute infections.
24	Folliculinum	Stimulate ovulation.
25	Gelsemium	Anti-viral, Neuro muscular affections, Heat stress.
26	Gloninum	Hyperemia, Sun Stroke.
27	Hamamelis	To prevent bleeding.
28	Hypericum	Anti-viral, Nerve Injuries, Induce CYP Enzymes.
29	Ignatia	Cannibalism
30	Iodum	Impaired Metabolism.
31	Kurchi	Dysenteries.
32	Lecithinum	Increase RBC, Galactagogues.
33	Lycopodium	Renal Health, Gout.
34	Merc solubilis	Ulcers, Coccidiosis, Syphilitic.
35	Natrum sulph	Avian Influenza.
36	Naja	Chronic Respiratory Diseases.
37	Nux vomica	Gastro-intestinal infections, Constipation, Polychrest
38	Mag Phos	Anti-muscular spasm, Torticollis.
39	Medicago Sativa	Weight gain.
40	Myrica Cerifera	Stimulate Hepatic filtration.
41	Ornithogalum	Inflamed GIT & Ulcers.
42	Pimpinella Ansium	Appetizer.
43	Pulsatilla	Synchronize the ovarian functions.
44	Pyrogenium	Septicemia.
45	Raphanus	Maintain rumen pH and Movements.

46	Rhus tox	Relieves joint pains.
47	Ruta	Reduces inflammatory edema.
48	Selenium	Sexual & Immune Health.
49	Silicia	Impaired Metabolism.
50	Sulphur	Impaired Nutrition, Cannibalism, Anti-psoric.
51	Symphytum	Helps in bone Re-union.
52	Thuja	Fowl pox, Bad effects of vaccinations. Respiratory illness.
53	Thymus Vulgaris	Immune modulator.
54	Verbascum Thalapsis	Broncho-dilator, Antimicrobial.
55	Veratrum album	Hyperemia, Prostrations, Greenish Diarrhea.
56	Veratrum viride	Sunstroke, Against diplococcus pneumonia.
57	Withania somnifera	Adaptogen.
58	Yucca	Kidney Health.
59	Zincum Met	Neurological and Immune weakness.
60	Zingiber officinalis	Action over GI Tract, Respiratory organs and Kidney.

Note: *In homeopathy, where individualization is key, a quick remedy profile acts as a valuable tool for both seasoned practitioners and those new to homeopathic medicine. It streamlines the process of remedy selection, ensuring accurate and effective treatment for individuals seeking homeopathic care.*

ESSENTIAL HOMEOPATHIC REMEDY PROFILES

1. **Aconitum napellus**
    - Source: Aconitum napellus is derived from the plant Aconitum, commonly known as monkshood or wolfsbane.
    - Preparation Method: The remedy is prepared using the roots of the plant through a specific dilution and succussion process.
    - Indications: Aconitum napellus is indicated in cases where fear, fright, chill, and exposure to cold, dry winds or excessive heat, especially from the sun, play a significant role. It is also relevant for instances of injury, surgical operations, shock, and catheter fever.
    - Key Symptoms: This remedy is characterized by the presence of great fear, anxiety, and worry accompanying every ailment. Additionally, it has the potential to slow down heart functions.
    - Constitutional Indications: While Aconitum napellus is considered a purely acute drug, it is most relevant in acute cases occurring in plethoric sanguine individuals. These individuals typically exhibit rigid fibers, dark hair and eyes, and are full of plethoric habits. The sedentary lifestyle of such individuals further accentuates the need for Aconitum.
    - Miasm: Psora is the predominant miasm associated with Aconitum napellus.

- Special Considerations: Aconitum is particularly relevant for strong, robust people and is the remedy of choice for rosy, chubby, and plethoric babies.
- Safety Data (1X): In terms of safety considerations, the use of Aconitum napellus in 1X potency may lead to agitations over blood circulation and potential irritation of brain functions. Monitoring and appropriate dosage are advised for safe usage.

2. **Arsenicum Album**
   - Indications and Uses: Arsenicum Album is a versatile homeopathic remedy known for its efficacy in addressing various health concerns, including.
   - Antiviral Properties: Effective against viral infections such as influenza (flu) and coronavirus (Corona).
   - Feverish Conditions: Indicated in cases of fever accompanied by great weakness and impaired nutrition.
   - Burning Pains: Provides relief from burning pains throughout the body, making it valuable for a range of discomforts.
   - Emergency Medicine: Essential in emergency situations, especially in cases of Status Asthmaticus and other life-threatening conditions.
   - Immune Modulator: Acts as an immune modulator, assisting the body in combating infections and enhancing overall immunity.
   - Respiratory Troubles: Beneficial for respiratory issues, offering relief in conditions such as asthma and other respiratory troubles.

- Prophylactic Use: Serves as a prophylactic medicine, particularly noted for its potential to prevent coronavirus infections.
- Septic Infections and Low Vitality: Effective against septic infections and conditions characterized by low vitality.
- Prevention of Acute Death: Known to prevent acute deaths, making it a crucial remedy in critical situations.
- Deep Acting Polychrest: A deep-acting polychrest, addressing a wide range of symptoms and constitutional aspects.
- Psychological Aspects: Useful for individuals with hypochondrial anxiety, characterized by excessive concerns about health.
- Aggravations: Symptoms worsen at night, in dusty environments, and after overeating fruits.
- Burning Sensation: Offers relief from burning sensations experienced throughout the body.
- Characteristic Discharges: Notable for greenish discharges in certain conditions.
- **Summary**

  Arsenicum Album emerges as a significant remedy with antiviral, immune-modulating, and emergency applications. It is indispensable in cases of respiratory troubles, septic infections, and situations where prevention of acute death is crucial. Additionally, its deep-acting nature and effectiveness against psychological symptoms make it a valuable component of homeopathic therapeutics.

3. **Bryonia Alba**

- Indications and Uses:
    - Acute Fever, Typhoid, Influenza: Indicated for acute febrile conditions, including typhoid and influenza, where fever is a prominent symptom.
    - Gastrointestinal Disorders: Beneficial for stomach and intestinal diseases, providing relief in cases of digestive disturbances.
    - Metabolic Disorders: Addressing metabolic disorders and promoting overall metabolic balance.
    - Infection Prevention: Useful as a preventive measure against infections, contributing to immune support.
    - Rheumatism:Effective in cases of rheumatism, particularly where symptoms manifest on the right side of the body.
- Psoric Miasm: Aligned with the psoric miasm, indicating its suitability for chronic and constitutional conditions.
- Constitutional: Suited for strong, healthy individuals with robust constitutions.
- Irritability: Helpful for conditions involving irritability and discomfort.
- Emetic Properties: Known for causing vomiting, making it applicable in cases where emesis is required.
- Dietary Preferences: Specific cravings for milk and soups, and a tendency to talk about business matters.
- Respiratory Conditions: Effective in addressing influenza, coryza, dryness of mucous membranes,

dehydration, dry cough, sore throat, asthma, and dyspnea.

- Musculoskeletal Issues: Beneficial for arthritis, with a tendency for symptoms to be worse on the right side.
- Headache and Constipation: Indicated for headaches associated with constipation, as well as vomiting. Symptoms worsen with motion.
- Therapeutics & Action
    - Fluid Retention: Has therapeutic effects on fluid retention issues.
    - Laxative Properties: Acts as a laxative, assisting in cases of constipation.
    - Emetic Effects: Exhibits emetic properties, useful in situations requiring induced vomiting.
- **Summary**

  Bryonia Alba emerges as a versatile homeopathic remedy with a broad spectrum of applications. It is particularly valuable in febrile conditions, gastrointestinal disorders, metabolic issues, and as a preventive measure against infections. Its affinity for the right side of the body, compatibility with the psoric miasm, and effectiveness in addressing both physical and mental symptoms contribute to its prominence in homeopathic therapeutics.

4. Calcarea Carbonica Ostrearum (Calcium Carbonate)

- Indications and Uses:
  - Enhancement of Normal Body Functions: Supports and enhances normal body functions, aiding in the patient's recovery from various illness stages.
  - Marked Remedy for Children: Particularly effective for children, addressing various health concerns common in this population.
  - Treatment of Low Blood Calcium Levels: Used to treat conditions associated with low blood calcium levels.
  - Osteoporosis and Osteomalacia/ Rickets: Indicated for osteoporosis and osteomalacia/rickets, conditions related to bone health.
  - Normocalcemic Primary Hyperparathyroidism (nPHPT): Addresses normocalcemic primary hyperparathyroidism, a disorder affecting the parathyroid glands.
  - Hypoparathyroidism: Useful in cases of hypoparathyroidism, a condition characterized by low levels of parathyroid hormone.
  - Pica: Addresses symptoms of pica, where individuals crave and consume non-food items.
- Miasm: Psoric miasm, indicating its suitability for chronic and constitutional conditions.
- Constitutional Type: Typically indicated for fair and plump individuals, especially those prone to boredom or lacking enthusiasm.

- Recovery from Illness: Particularly beneficial for individuals who tend to get sick easily and take a prolonged time to recover from illnesses.
- Great Constitutional & Intercurrent Remedy: Considered a great constitutional and intercurrent remedy, offering broad-spectrum support.
- Physical Symptoms: Profuse perspiration, especially on the head. Malnourished children with weak bones. Sensitivity to cold.
- Dietary Cravings: Craving for eggs and a tendency to eat non-food items (pica).
- Digestive Symptoms: Heartburn and upset stomach.Constipation.
- Other General Symptoms: Weight loss and anorexia. Insomnia and fatigue. Inattention.
- Safety Data (1X): Constipation and upset stomach may occur in some cases.Possible allergic reactions like rash, itching, and swelling (over the face, tongue, and throat). Overdose may lead to weight loss.
- **Summary**

  Calcarea Carbonica Ostrearum stands out as a versatile homeopathic remedy with a focus on enhancing normal body functions and supporting recovery. Its applications range from addressing children's health issues to treating conditions related to bone health and calcium levels. As a constitutional remedy, it proves beneficial for individuals with specific physical and psychological characteristics, making it a valuable addition to homeopathic therapeutics. Safety considerations include potential digestive symptoms and allergic reactions in some instances.

5. **Calendula Officinalis**

- Indications and Uses:
    - Lymphatic Disorders: Effective in the treatment of both primary and secondary lymphedema, promoting lymphatic system health.
    - Chronic Venous Insufficiency: Indicated for chronic venous insufficiency, aiding in venous circulation.
    - Post-Traumatic Edema: Useful in addressing edema resulting from trauma, supporting post-traumatic recovery.
    - Enhancement of MLD Therapy: Enhances the results of Manual Lymph Drainage (MLD) therapy, contributing to improved lymphatic function.
    - Heat Stress: Provides relief in conditions related to heat stress, both internally and externally.
    - Dermatological Conditions: External application for various dermatological conditions, including wounds, injuries, cracks, dermatitis (irritant contact, allergic, dry eczema, seborrheic, neuro, and stasis).
    - Prickly Heat: Alleviates symptoms associated with prickly heat.
    - Oral Health: Beneficial for mouth ulcers, tooth decay, and bad breath.
    - Wound Healing: External applications for injuries, wounds, lacerated wounds, and warts, aiding in the healing process.

  - Antiseptic, Antiviral, Antibacterial:Exhibits antiseptic, antiviral, and antibacterial properties, contributing to infection control.
  - Hepatic Protector: Acts as a hepatic protector, supporting liver health.
  - Anti-Inflammatory and Antipyretic: Has anti-inflammatory and antipyretic effects, addressing inflammation and fever.
- Physiological Actions: Stimulates lymphatic drainage. Reduces the reverse transcription ability of viruses. Promotes a response from natural killer cells. Acts as an elastase and collagenase inhibitor.
- Safety Data (1X): External use may cause very minimal skin irritations.
- **Summary**

  Calendula Officinalis is a versatile homeopathic remedy with a broad range of applications. From addressing lymphatic disorders to dermatological conditions and oral health, its diverse therapeutic effects make it valuable in various medical contexts. Additionally, its physiological actions contribute to infection control and immune system support. Safety considerations primarily involve minimal skin irritations with external use.

6. **Capsicum Annum**

- Indications and Uses
    - ➢ Arthritis and Chronic Pains: Effective in addressing arthritis and chronic pains, providing relief from discomfort.
    - ➢ Nerve Damages and Neuropathies: Indicated for nerve damages, diabetic neuropathy, and nerve damage caused by conditions like shingles (postherpetic neuralgia).
    - ➢ Scarlet Fever: Used in cases of scarlet fever, aiding in symptom relief.
    - ➢ Mucous Membrane Action: Acts on mucous membranes, providing therapeutic benefits.
    - ➢ Alternative to Antibiotic Growth Promoters: Considered a promising alternative to antibiotic growth promoters due to its high content of bioactive substances.
- Antiviral Properties: Exhibits antiviral properties, contributing to immune system support.
- Research on Poultry Health: Research indicates potential benefits against Newcastle Disease Virus (NDV) in poultry, impacting antibody response and improving meat quality.
- Immune Response Enhancement: Enhances immune response to infectious bronchitis disease and infectious bursa disease.
- Diathesis, Dyspepsia, and Gout: Addresses plethoric diathesis, home sickness, gout, and dyspepsia accompanied by flatulence.
- Burning Pains and Tympanitis: Effective in cases of burning pains, tympanitis (inflammation of the

abdominal cavity), and earaches with pus discharges.

- Urethral Pains, Back Pain, and Neuralgias: Provides relief from urethral pains, back pain, and neuralgias following shingles and herpes infections.
- Cluster Headache: Alleviates cluster headaches with intense pain around one eye, especially at night.
- Physiological Activity: Selective impairment of pain (C-type) fibers, affecting pain sensation from the abdominal viscera to the central nervous system (CNS).
- Therapeutic Actions (1X to 12X): Stimulation of the gastrointestinal tract (GIT). Inhibition of the development of pathogenic bacteria.
- Anti-coccidial properties. Antiviral agent impacting T cells and cytokine production.
- Safety Data (1X): Long-term use and overdosing may cause irritation, sweating, and a runny nose.
- **Summary**

  Capsicum Annum, with its diverse range of applications, proves valuable in addressing various health issues, from pain management to immune system support. Its potential as an alternative to antibiotics in poultry health and its impact on physiological pain fibers make it an intriguing component of homeopathic therapeutics. As with any remedy, caution should be exercised regarding potential irritations and adverse effects with prolonged use or overdosing.

7. Carbo Vegetabilis

- Indications and Uses
  - Gastritis and Respiratory Acidosis: Indicated for gastritis and respiratory acidosis, particularly in cases of status asthmaticus.
  - Status Asthmaticus: Effective in managing status asthmaticus, a severe and potentially life-threatening form of asthma.
  - Imperfect Oxidation and Toxemia Prevention: Addresses imperfect oxidation, helping to improve vitality and prevent toxemia.
  - Detoxification: Acts as a detoxifier, aiding in the removal of toxins from the body, particularly from urea.
  - Renal Support: Assists the kidneys in filtering residues of drugs and toxins, promoting renal health.
  - Gastrointestinal Symptoms: Alleviates flatulence, abdominal pain, cramps, and helps rebalance the acid-base balance of the respiratory system during status asthmaticus.
  - Respiratory Distress: Indicated in cases of slight pulse, oppressed chest with dyspnea, and weakness in patients experiencing respiratory distress.
- Constitutional Characteristics: Suited for individuals who are sluggish, fatigued, lazy, and have a tendency towards chronic complaints.
- Residual Effects of Previous Illness: Effective for those who never fully recovered from previous illnesses, addressing lingering symptoms.

- Cyanosis and Lowered Vital Power: Addresses conditions where the body becomes blue, icy cold, with lowered vital power and loss of vital fluids after drugging.
- Physiological Activity: Functions as a detoxifier and promotes intestinal functions.
- **Summary**

  Carbo Vegetabilis emerges as a versatile homeopathic remedy, particularly beneficial for gastrointestinal and respiratory issues. Its ability to address imperfect oxidation, prevent toxemia, and support detoxification makes it valuable in various clinical contexts. Additionally, it is well-suited for individuals who exhibit constitutional characteristics of sluggishness, chronicity, and lingering effects from previous illnesses. The remedy's physiological actions align with detoxification and promoting intestinal functions. Careful consideration of individual symptoms and constitutional traits is essential for its effective use in homeopathic practice.

8. Chamomilla

- Indications and Uses:
  - Acute Conditions: Indicated for various acute conditions, providing relief in situations of sudden onset.
  - Muscle Spasms and Painful Contractions: Effective in alleviating muscle spasms, cramps, and painful contractions or tightening of muscles.
  - Gastrointestinal Inflammatory Disorders: Useful in gastrointestinal inflammatory disorders, addressing symptoms such as dyspepsia, abdominal colics, upset stomach, and GERD in its early stages.
  - Menstrual Complaints: Helpful in managing menstrual complaints, providing relief from associated discomfort.
  - Motion Sickness: Addresses symptoms of motion sickness, offering relief from nausea and vomiting.
  - Chemotherapy-Induced Mucositis: Effective in managing chemotherapy-induced mucositis, a condition characterized by inflammation of the mucous membranes.
  - Painful Conditions: Indicated for intolerable pain during muscle spasms, cramps, and painful contractions, with amelioration through vomiting.
  - Spasmodic Pains: Relieves spasmodic pains aggravated by nausea, flatulence, and vomiting.

    - Toothache: Provides relief from toothache and associated symptoms.
- Pediatric Ailments: Suitable for irritable children and crying children with gastrointestinal ailments, constipation, and teething issues.
- Physiological Activity: Exhibits anti-inflammatory, analgesic, antipyretic, and emetic properties.
- Therapeutic Actions (1X to 12X)
    - Escalates gastroesophageal emptying. Helps in the symptomatic treatment of gastrointestinal problems.
    - Mild blood-thinning effects.
- Safety Data (1X)
    - Possible allergic reactions and hypersensitivity.
    - Avoid use in pregnant ladies.
    - Caution required with blood thinners, Allium sativa, Ginko biloba, Hypericum, Valeriana officinalis, and Serenoa repens.
- **Summary**

  Chamomilla is a versatile homeopathic remedy known for its effectiveness in acute conditions, particularly those involving pain, spasms, and gastrointestinal disturbances. It demonstrates therapeutic actions that range from anti-inflammatory and analgesic effects to aiding in gastroesophageal emptying. While it is generally safe, caution is advised regarding potential allergic reactions and contraindications with certain medications and herbs. Chamomilla's application is wide-ranging, making it a valuable component in addressing various acute health issues.

9. Coffea Cruda

- Indications and Uses:
  - Insomnia: Indicated for insomnia, especially in cases where the mind is overactive and sleep is elusive.
  - Neurological Troubles: Effective in addressing various neurological troubles, providing relief from associated symptoms.
  - Skin Diseases and Intolerance of Pains: Used for skin diseases and conditions where there is an intolerance to pain.
  - Ailments from Sudden Mental Emotions: Helpful in cases where ailments arise from sudden and intense mental emotions.
  - Restlessness and Sensitivity: Effective for individuals who are restless, highly sensitive, and easily affected by their surroundings.
  - Trio Painful Remedy: Part of the trio of painful remedies along with Aconite and Chamomilla, especially when intense pain is a prominent symptom.
  - Physiological Activity:Exhibits anti-sycotic, hypnotic, analgesic, and anxiolytic properties.
- Suited for Specific Physical Characteristics: Suited for thin, tall individuals with a black complexion, chloretic and sanguine temperament, and a predisposition to uric acid diathesis.

- Therapeutic Actions (1X to 12X):
  - ➢ Beneficial in Attention Deficit Hyperactivity Disorder (ADHD).
  - ➢ Effective in addressing neuralgic pains, including cephalalgia (headaches) and toothaches.
  - ➢ Acts as an anti-stress remedy.
- Safety Data (1X): Prolonged continuous usage may lead to masking of actual signs and symptoms of body impairments.

  Summary: Coffea Cruda is a homeopathic remedy primarily used for conditions related to sleep, neurological troubles, and skin diseases. It is well-suited for individuals with specific physical characteristics and temperament. The remedy's effectiveness extends to addressing ailments triggered by sudden mental emotions and providing relief in cases of heightened sensitivity and restlessness. It is important to consider the safety data, especially the caution against prolonged continuous usage, to ensure its appropriate and effective application in homeopathic practice.

10. Pulsatilla Nigricans

- Indications and Uses:
  - Menstrual Irregularities: Indicated for all kinds of menstrual irregularities, addressing various symptoms related to the menstrual cycle.
  - Dermatological Disorders:
  - Effective in treating dermatological disorders such as boils and papules.
  - Teething Issues: Beneficial for teething issues in infants, providing relief from associated symptoms.
  - Back Pain and Sciatica:
  - Used for back pain, sciatica, and labor pain.
  - Yellowish Green Discharges: Addresses conditions with yellowish-green discharges.
  - Asthmatic Troubles:
  - Effective in cases of asthmatic troubles, providing relief from respiratory symptoms.
  - Reproductive Dysfunctions:
  - Treats reproductive dysfunctions, premenstrual syndrome, and chronic epididymitis.
  - Fever and Tension Headaches:
  - Used for fever and tension headaches.
  - Migraine and Insomnia:
  - Indicated for migraine and insomnia, especially related to emotional states.
  - Emotional Characteristics:
  - Ailments from jealousy, childishness, and consolation ameliorates symptoms.

- Thirstless and tends to take a long time to fall asleep, sometimes trying to sleep with open eyes.

- Female Remedy: Considered a prominent remedy for female-related issues.
- Emotional Expression: Expresses emotions openly, with a tendency for weeping.
- Irritability and Dominating Behavior: Exhibits irritability and may display dominating behavior.
- Miasm and Temperament: Psoric and sycotic miasm with phlegmatic temperaments.
- Dietary Preferences: Aversion to meat, butter, fat food, and milk. Desire for alcoholic drinks.
- Hyperactive States and Opposition Tendencies: Tends to be hyperactive and may have a tendency to oppose others.
- Respiratory Symptoms: Cough with dry, allergic symptoms, catarrhal conditions, and yellowish thick mucus.
- Testicle Pain and Tenderness:
- Addresses testicle pain and tenderness, usually on one side.
- Physiological Activity: Exhibits antioxidant, anticancer, cytotoxic, and antipsychotic properties.
- Safety Data (1X):
    - Misuse can lead to various symptoms, including diarrhea, vomiting, convulsions, hypotension, and coma.
    - Contact with the skin can cause rash, inflammation, and itching.
    - Ingestion may cause allergic reactions, irritate the nose, eyes, mouth, and throat.

- Should not be taken during pregnancy or lactation.

- **Summary:**

  Pulsatilla Nigricans is a versatile homeopathic remedy with a broad spectrum of applications. It is prominently used for menstrual irregularities, reproductive dysfunctions, emotional disturbances, and respiratory issues. The remedy's physiological activities extend to antioxidant, anticancer, cytotoxic, and antipsychotic properties. However, caution is advised regarding safety, especially the potential adverse effects and contraindications, particularly during pregnancy and lactation. Individualized assessment of symptoms and constitutional characteristics is crucial for effective application in homeopathic practice.

Conclusion Note

The culmination of "Poultry Homeopathy: Advancing Homeopathic Research in Poultry Healthcare" marks a significant stride in the integration of homeopathic principles into the realm of poultry health. This comprehensive exploration delves into the intricate balance between traditional practices and modern advancements, reshaping the landscape of poultry healthcare.

Key Takeaways

- Homeopathy's Evolution: The book charts the evolution of homeopathy in the context of poultry health, emphasizing its adaptability to modern research and technological revolutions.
- Holistic Poultry Care: Through detailed discussions on various diseases, the book underscores the holistic nature of homeopathic solutions, addressing not only symptoms but the underlying imbalances that contribute to poultry health challenges.
- Research Insights: It delves into the latest research findings, shedding light on how homeopathy aligns with contemporary scientific understanding, offering evidence-based insights into its efficacy.

- Challenges and Opportunities: The book candidly explores the challenges faced in adopting homeopathy in poultry healthcare, offering a roadmap to overcome skepticism and foster acceptance. It positions homeopathy not as a replacement but as a complementary approach.
- Sustainable Poultry Farming: Central to the narrative is the role of homeopathy in promoting sustainable poultry farming practices. It addresses concerns such as antibiotic resistance, residue build-up, and the broader impact of conventional methods on the environment.
- Call for Collaboration: The concluding chapters extend a call for collaboration between traditional veterinary practices and homeopathy, fostering an environment where both can coexist and contribute to the well-being of poultry.
- Looking Forward: As the book reaches its conclusion, it opens the door for further exploration, urging practitioners, researchers, and stakeholders to continue advancing the integration of homeopathy in poultry healthcare. The journey outlined in this book is not an endpoint but a catalyst for ongoing dialogue, research, and innovation in redefining the future of poultry health through the lens of homeopathy.

Dr Muhammed KS, BHMS

POULTRY HOMEOPATHY

"Advancing Homeopathic Research in Poultry Healthcare"

2nd Edition

INDEX

BIBILIOGRAPHY

- *Homeopathic Materia Medica with Repertory, William Boricke.*
- *The Merck Veterinary Manual.*
- *Vethomeopath. Dr. Surjith Singh Makker*
- *Kent Materia Medica*
- *Encyclopedia of Homeopathy, DR. Andrew Lockie. DK Publishers.*
- *Duke's Phytochemical and Ethnobotanical Database.*
- *An introduction to pharmacists-Homeopathic medicines, Christopher. R. Marville. D.*
- *Poultry Homeopathy. Dr. B.P Madrewar. 2nd Edition-2007.*
- *The poultry doctor, Borricke and Taffel.*
- *Encyclopedia Of Homeopathic Pharmacopoeia of Drug Index. Dr. P.N Varma and Dr. Indu Vaid. - 2017, B.jain Publishers.*
- *Homeopathic pharmacopoeia, M.Bhattacharya.Principles and practice of homeopathy, Dr. David Owen.*
- *Text book of homeopathic pharmacy, Mandal and Mandal.*
- *Ncbi.nlm.nih.gov*
- *Google.com*
- *National Journal of Homeopathy.*
- *Asian journal of Homeopathy.*
- *European Journal of Classical Homeopathy*
- *American Journal of Homeopathic Medicine*
- *British Homeopathic journal*
- *Pubmed.ncbi.nlm.nih.com*
- *Msdpoultryvetmanual.com.*
- *The poultrysite.com*
- *Europepmc.org*
- *Chatgpt.com*
- *Resaerchgate.net*
- *Bioline.com*
- *Healthline.com*
- *Biomin.net*
- *www.Similima.com*
- *Bahvs.com*
- *Nopr.niscair.res.in*
- *Cfsph.iastate.edu*
- *Mehakwellnesscentre.com*
- *Cimsasia.com*
- *Bimecentral.com*
- *www.stgeorgehomeopathy.com*

AUTHOR PROFILE

Dr. Muhammed KS is a highly skilled medical professional with over 7+ years of diverse experience in healthcare. He excels in various aspects such as product development, advanced product quality enhancement, and antibiotic replacement projects focused on poultry. His expertise extends to business development and collaboration, making him a notable figure in the field.

Dr. Muhammed KS has successfully acquired several Qualifications and certifications, showcasing his commitment to continuous learning and professional development:

- ✓ **Advance Product Quality Planning & New Product Development.**
  Certification from Confederation of Indian Quality Institute, Bangalore.
- ✓ **FOSTAC.**
  Certifications from The Food Safety and Standards Authority of India (FSSAI).
- ✓ **Public Health Nutrition.**
  Institute of Health Management Research
- ✓ **Basic Research Methodology.**
  Research Skill Development Academy, Mangalore
- ✓ **Health Emergency Programme.**
  Health care operation planning and Guidelines - WHO.
- ✓ **Nano Medicine Treatment Protocol.**
  National Institute of Technology, Calicut.
- ✓ **Bio-Nano Medicine,**
  Make intern Institute, Bangalore.

- ✓ **Nano Homeopathica.**
  Scientific Research, Vinayaka Missions University, Salem.
- ✓ **Malligma Banerji Protocols for Life Threatening Diseases.**
  IHK, Kerala.
- ✓ **Case Report Writing,**
  RIH, Kerala.

Dr. Muhammed KS's extensive knowledge and diverse skill set make him an extraordinary author contributing valuable insights to the publication book.

His significant contributions to the published works, "POULTRY HOMEOPATHY-Scope of Homeopathic Research in Poultry, First Edition" and "POULTRY HOMEOPATHY - Advancing Homeopathic Research in Poultry Healthcare - 2nd Edition," have established him as a thought leader in the field of homeopathic research for poultry healthcare. These books serve as invaluable resources, providing insights and advancements in poultry health management.

As Dr. Muhammed KS ventures into the upcoming book, "MODERN HOMEOPATHICA - New Homeopathic Conceptualization, 1st Edition," there is anticipation for groundbreaking ideas and a fresh perspective on homeopathic practices. With his exceptional knowledge and dedication to advancing healthcare through homeopathy, this upcoming publication promises to be a milestone in the realm of homeopathic literature.

Dr. Muhammed KS's journey exemplifies a commitment to pushing the boundaries of knowledge in poultry health, and his works continue to be a source of inspiration for researchers, practitioners, and enthusiasts.

Upcoming Publications
Prior Booking Offer: 20% Discount
Call Us: 6374 1616 84

PRESCRIPTIONs

HOMEOPATHIC DERMATOLOGY

Dr. Mathew Jacob, BHMS

1st Edition

MODERN HOMEOPATHICA

New Homeopathic Conceptualization
Dr. Muhammed KS, BHMS

1st Edition

My Health Guide Publications
Razi Health Care Initiatives

www.myhealthguide2022@gmail.com
My Health Guide Publications | 2024

📚 Explore the Future of Health Literature! 🌿

Embark on a transformative journey with our upcoming health publications: "PRESCRIPTIONs: Homeopathic Dermatology" and "MODERN HOMEOPATHICA: New Homeopathic Conceptualization." 📘✨

🖊 Calling All Writers and Health Enthusiasts!

Your words can shape the narrative of holistic healthcare. Join us in crafting narratives that blend homeopathic wisdom with modern understanding. Whether you're a seasoned writer or an aspiring wordsmith, this is your chance to contribute to a literary revolution in health.

✨ Why Contribute?

Influence the future of homeopathic literature.
Illuminate the pages with your unique perspective.
Inspire practitioners and enthusiasts worldwide.
Be a part of the holistic health movement.

🌐 How to Contribute?

Submit Your Work: Share your articles, case studies, or insights related to Health Care.

- Be a Part of Transformation: Your words have the power to transform perspectives and elevate understanding. Be a guiding light in the world of holistic health.
- Connect and Collaborate: Join a community of like-minded writers and health enthusiasts. Collaborate with professionals and contribute to a shared vision of holistic well-being.

📩 Submit Your Contribution:

myhealthguide2022@gmail.com

- 🔜 Stay Tuned for the Book Launch! Your contribution will be part of a groundbreaking publication that redefines health literature. Let your words echo in the minds of readers seeking a holistic approach to well-being.

✍️📖 #Health Literature # Homeopathic# Writers Wanted

🌿 Join Us on this Literary Adventure!

Call Us: 6374 1616 84 | myhealthguide2022@gmail.com My Health Guide Publications | Malappuram | Kerala-676552

PRESCRIPTIONs

Homeopathic Dermatology

Dr. Mathew Jacob, BHMS - 1st Edition

Embark on a comprehensive exploration of dermatology through the lens of homeopathy with Dr. Mathew Jacob's upcoming book. In this 1st Edition, Dr. Jacob delves into the intricate connections between homeopathic principles and dermatological conditions. With a blend of theoretical insights and practical applications, the book promises to be a valuable resource for both practitioners and enthusiasts. Stay tuned for a holistic journey into the world of Homeopathic Dermatology.

MODERN HOMEOPATHICA

New Homeopathic Conceptualization

By Dr. Muhammed KS, BHMS - 1st Edition

Explore the future of homeopathy with "Modern Homeopathica," a groundbreaking book. This visionary work introduces innovative conceptualizations in homeopathy, offering fresh perspectives and advanced approaches to homeopathic practice. Driven by extensive research and practical insights, the book promises to be a game-changer in the realm of homeopathic medicine. Stay tuned for an enlightening journey into the modern evolution of homeopathy.

As we present these two compelling additions to the homeopathic literature, we invite you to delve into the realms of Homeopathic Dermatology and the Modern Evolution of Homeopathy.

"PRESCRIPTIONs" and "MODERN HOMEOPATHICA" promise not only to expand your knowledge but also to revolutionize your approach to homeopathic practice. Whether you are a seasoned practitioner seeking advanced insights or an enthusiast eager to explore the future of homeopathy, these editions are designed to be your trusted companions on this enlightening journey. Stay tuned for an enriching experience that transcends conventional boundaries and ushers in a new era in homeopathic understanding and application.

www.ingramcontent.com/pod-product-compliance
Lightning Source LLC
LaVergne TN
LVHW061545070526
838199LV00077B/6908

* 9 7 8 9 3 6 2 6 1 6 4 2 5 *